GROCERY MAKEOVER

SMALL CHANGES FOR BIG RESULTS

Julie Feldman, MPH, RD

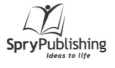

SpryPublishing
ideas to life

This edition is published by Spry Publishing LLC
2500 South State Street
Ann Arbor, MI 48104 USA

Printed and bound in the United States.

10 9 8 7 6 5 4 3 2 1

Library of Congress Control Number: 2013930271

Paperback ISBN: 978-1-938170-17-1
E-book ISBN: 978-1-938170-18-8

Disclaimer: Spry Publishing LLC does not assume responsibility
for the contents or opinions expressed herein. Although every precaution
is taken to ensure that information is accurate as of the date of publication,
differences of opinion exist. The opinions expressed herein are those of
the author and do not necessarily reflect the views of the publisher.
The information contained in this book is not intended to replace
professional advisement of an individual's doctor prior to beginning
or changing an individual's course of treatment.

Information in this publication was accurate, to the best of our knowledge,
at the time of printing. However, web sites are subject to change, and we
encourage the reader to confirm with additional sources of information.

THIS BOOK IS DEDICATED
to all of the people and places in my life that have taught, loved, motivated, trusted, cherished, and inspired me along my path. To the University of Michigan for giving me my education and my husband, Go Blue! To my parents—both those who gave birth to me (Dennis and Ellen) and those whom I have gained along my way (Mort, Millie, Cheryl, and Paul)—who are my biggest cheerleaders and whose unconditional love has taught me to believe that anything is possible. To my children Emily, Allison, and Robert, who inspire me each and every day to learn new things and see the goodness in the world. To my husband, Brad, who not only was my first great English teacher, but who has stood by my side through every grown-up obstacle and whose deep love is the fuel that feeds me each and every day. To my incredible network of friends and extended family, whose excitement for this project and all that I do amazes me. Specifically, Amy, Seth, Danny, Michael, Lori, Jake, Randi, Steve, Sammy, Ariel, Ryann, Rebecca, Jessie, Heather, Franci, Sam, Eden, Kevin, Melissa, Marty, Robyn, Mitch, Lezlie, Eric, Melissa, Jeremy, Alisa, Mark, Erin, and Glenn. To my clients who practice the principles of this book each and every day and whose determination and success are a true inspiration.

This book is also dedicated to all of its readers; especially the ones who have always wanted to live a healthy life and just didn't know how to do it. Whoever would have thought this overweight teenager would grow up to write a book on healthy eating and shopping? Whether you are 8 or 80, it is okay to prioritize your health and make good choices when it comes to food. One day at a time, you can realize your true potential.

Contents

Preface

As a mother of three young children, our daily family schedule has me racing in many different directions. From PTO meetings to dance class, to basketball and baseball, our lives are so hectic that even the necessary things like grocery shopping are challenging to fit in. And let's say you do find the time to make it to the market—what on earth are you supposed to purchase? For most consumers, it's the foods they know their family will eat with minimal complaints or the sale items that fit into the family budget that make it into the grocery cart each week. Because of all the constraints on each of us, fueling our families well has become quite the challenge of the modern day household.

Thankfully, for my family, I have a Master's Degree in human nutrition and have been a practicing dietitian for 14 years. I therefore know what to buy at a grocery store to ensure that my family and I are eating well. However, it's pretty easy to understand how mindless eating and grocery shopping are almost a given in many households with exhausting and stressful schedules. Grocery shopping is perhaps one of the most mundane errands we run. Walking through the doors of the market several times a week, it hardly seems the spiritual gateway for a health transformation. What I hope you will learn from reading this book, however, is that the market is our passage to good health. There is truly no other place we visit that has more to do with how we feel, act, and live.

You, as the chief grocery shopper in your household, make decisions regarding the quality and quantity of products and, thus, impact how your family lives. With nearly 40,000 traditional grocery stores throughout the United States, each one housing nearly 60,000 different items, learning how to grocery shop in a healthy way is a necessity if your goal is to nourish and raise a healthy family. This process, which seems overwhelming, truly boils down to having basic nutrition knowledge. I'm not referring to the latest diet trend or celebrity weight loss scheme, but rather to basic biology and chemistry, which is a bit less cool but a lot more practical. It also requires reading and understanding product labels, which include ingredient lists and federally allowed health claims that appear on the foods we purchase.

As a registered dietitian, I have the awesome job of helping people live their healthiest lives. The people who seek me out are contemplating making necessary changes to their diet in hopes of feeling well, looking good, and becoming healthier versions of themselves. We all recognize that change, albeit often necessary, is one of the most difficult processes to endure. The change required to achieve good health is a significant transformation for many people. My goal in counseling my clients is to help them develop a healthy relationship between their bodies and food. This requires dedication and introspection. The connection that we have with food is deeply rooted and far-reaching. It often dates back to our earliest childhood memories and is completely entwined with our emotions. The fact is that I spend about 90 percent of my time with my clients talking about their feelings and emotions and only about 10 percent talking about food. That being said, you can't make good choices about food without knowing how certain foods and ingredients can affect your health and emotional well-being.

There are many books about health and wellness (a whole section in the bookstore, in fact). But just because you know the concepts of eating healthy does not mean you are able to translate that into real life. I studied biology in graduate school but I'm not whipping up vaccines in my kitchen sink! When it comes to diet, recommendations need to be specific and applicable. True success in the area of eating healthy can be measured by biological alterations including weight changes, cholesterol levels, vitamin levels, need for medications, and overall quality of life improvements. By better understanding the nutritional value behind the foods for which we shop, true health changes will be attained.

The favorite part of my job is watching my clients reap the

rewards of their positive lifestyle changes. This happens not simply because they are eating spinach and flaxseeds. It happens because they are educated on how certain foods make them feel great or lousy. It happens because they become more peaceful in each moment they make a choice about food. With this level of confidence, the cravings to have certain less healthy foods are far surpassed by their desire to achieve the emotional high that comes with feeling great about themselves. I am excited to be a part of your transformation to better health as you seek guidance from this book in a very practical way.

Part One
Getting Started

The Basics of Sound Nutrition

Nelson Mandela once said, "Education is the most powerful weapon which you can use to change the world." This could not be truer than in the instance of diet and wellness. The process of learning about food and its effects on our body has the ability to change who we are as consumers and caregivers to our families. In order to read labels and become an educated grocery consumer, you must have a crash course in Nutrition 101.

To uncover the mystery of nutritional science and discover practical and easy-to-understand food facts, we must begin at the macronutrient level. The foods that we eat can be divided into three main macronutrients. They are carbohydrates, proteins, and fats. Each of these are digested, absorbed, and utilized differently by our bodies.

Over the years, numerous theories have been developed concerning which type of fuel is better for us, or which one we should limit or eliminate in order to achieve good health. These are the low-fat, low-carb, high-protein diets you've undoubtedly heard of. The fact is that our bodies need all three types of nourishment! Furthermore, how we eat and combine these macronutrients can be the key to feeling great and maintaining a healthy weight.

Carbohydrates

The majority of our diet is comprised of carbohydrates (carbs). Most health-governing agencies recommend that carbs make up around 50 percent of our daily intake. Carbs, by definition, are sugars and their derivatives. Carbs in real life are a large food group that includes breads, cereals, grains, crackers, pasta, rice, cookies, candy, cakes, fruits, vegetables, and dairy products. Carbohydrates can be broken down into monosaccharides, disaccharides, and polysaccharides.

Monosaccharides are simple sugars such as glucose. Glucose, fructose, galactose, xylose, and ribose are all sugars in their simplest forms. When they are combined together they make disaccharides. For example, glucose + galactose = lactose, the sugar we find in milk and dairy products. Glucose + glucose = maltose or malt sugar, and glucose + fructose = sucrose, which is what we find in table sugar. Taking this math lesson one step further, polysaccharides are the result of even longer chains of monosaccharides being linked. Polysaccharides include starches and dietary fiber.

Many food producers aim to make their products seem healthier by using catchphrases such as "sweetened with honey" instead of just saying sugar. They hope that you do not realize that honey is made out of something called invert sugar (modified sucrose). This is just one of many ways by which food labels and packaging can be confusing. Similarly, you may see a product that boasts that it is "sweetened with fruit juice." That food producer hopes you do not know that fruit juice is comprised almost entirely of fructose. The bottom line is that sugar is sugar, and, for the most part, the way our bodies handle sugar in all of its forms is very similar.

As a dietitian, I think of carbohydrates fitting into one of two categories—fiber-less and fiber-full. The fiber-less group is made up of refined or processed carbohydrates. This includes everything from cheesy crackers to potato chips, sugary cereals to white bread, candy to sweetened beverages. Refined carbohydrates are those that have been processed to such an extent that the healthful qualities associated with the food they are made from have been lost. When we choose these foods, they are digested and absorbed very quickly in the small intestine, creating a spike in our blood sugar. This sudden increase in blood sugar generates an equal production of a hormone in our body called insulin. Insulin, produced by the pancreas, is a fat-storage hormone.

Eating a concentrated sweet or refined carbohydrate on its own causes a spike in your blood sugar. This is sort of like a party that gets out of control, and we all know what happens when a party gets out of control—the police come. The police in this case is insulin. The officers pick up all the offenders (blood sugar) who are having a party and they drive them home. Some sugar will be stored in our muscles in the form of glycogen, while some will find haven in our liver. The remaining blood sugar that needs a place to stay will find shelter in our fat cells. This process of raising our blood sugar quickly, high levels of insulin production, and the subsequent fat storage and falling blood sugars is dangerous.

Parents and children alike can typically relate to this scenario by thinking about the "after-school snack." Most kids will come home from school starving and choose a refined carbohydrate. Whether it's pretzels or cookies, these foods create about 30 minutes of satisfaction followed by the child saying, "I'm still hungry!" For many people, this pattern of eating takes place throughout the entire day, resulting in constant feelings of hunger and lethargy (we are tired when our blood sugar is too high or too low). In addition, people experience unnecessary weight gain.

When We Eat...

insulin

blood sugar

Fiber less carbohydrate

When we eat carbohyrate foods that don't have fiber when we are hungry, they cause a spike in our blood sugar. Spikes in blood sugar are associated with excess fat storage and constant feelings of hunger and cravings.

hungry

hungry

1/2 hour

Sugar Content of Some Common Snack Foods/Beverages

Food	Sugar (g)
12-ounce soda	39
Regular Snickers bar	30
1 bag Skittles	47
1 Fruit-by-the-Foot	10
Powerbar	23
2 Hostess Twinkies	37
Yoplait yogurt	27
12-ounce McFlurry with Oreo Cookies	73
2 Pop-Tarts	34
Cinnamon roll	55
Starbucks' Grande Mocha Frappuccino with whipped cream	47

The second category of carbohydrates is the fiber-full group. Here we are talking about whole grains, fruits and vegetables, beans, lentils, and popcorn. I know the first group sounds a lot more fun, but learning how to select, cook, and enjoy the fiber-full carbohydrates is just pages away! When deciding which foods to shop for and provide for your family, choosing mostly fiber-full carbohydrates is the way to go. Fiber extends many benefits to our overall health and quality of life. In my usual one-hour consultations with clients, we spend at least 15 minutes talking about fiber—it's that important! Fiber is unique in that it is the only nutrient that we eat that we don't break down and absorb. In our small intestine, which is where most digestion and absorption take place, fiber ensures that these processes are slow and deliberate. In contrast to the

Ideal Blood Sugars

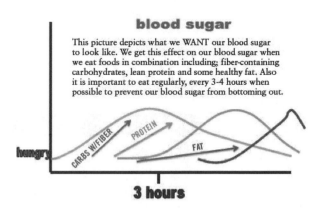

blood sugar

This picture depicts what we WANT our blood sugar to look like. We get this effect on our blood sugar when we eat foods in combination including; fiber-containing carbohydrates, lean protein and some healthy fat. Also it is important to eat regularly, every 3-4 hours when possible to prevent our blood sugar from bottoming out.

hungry

CARBS W/FIBER

PROTEIN

FAT

3 hours

first illustration, when we choose foods that contain adequate amounts of fiber, our blood sugar does not spike quickly. Think of fiber as a security guard, allowing only one molecule of sugar to be absorbed at a time. This creates a slow and steady source of energy for our bodies that does not cause a large production of insulin. When we eat this way throughout the day we feel great. We have energy, lack cravings, and are more likely to be more physically active. An important first step in your grocery transition is making the shift from fiber-less to fiber-full carbohydrates. But carbohydrates are just one piece of the puzzle.

Age	Fiber Grams Needed Per Day
Children 0–20	Add 5 to age to figure daily goal (e.g., a 5 year old needs at least 10 g/day)
Adults	25–35 grams

Protein

The second macronutrient your body needs daily is protein. Protein is comprised of amino acids. Protein can be found in foods such as meat, poultry, fish, egg whites, dairy products, beans, tofu, and nuts. While we used to think of amino acids as simply the building blocks of lean muscle mass, current science is exploring a whole myriad of ways that proteins influence our overall health. Proteins are composed of 21 different amino acids. Of these 21, 9 are referred to as essential amino acids as the human body is unable to synthesize them on its own and they must be obtained from the diet.

Not all protein foods are created equal for the purposes of tissue regeneration and muscle development. Proteins are graded on a quality scale called the PDCAAS (Protein Digestibility Corrected Amino Acid Score). This scale takes into account the quality and quantity of amino acids in a specific food, as well as the need for those amino acids by the human body. Four foods have a perfect 1.0 PDCAAS score, namely egg white, casein and whey (milk proteins), and soy protein. Other proteins, such as beef (0.92), nuts (0.52), and wheat (0.42), lack one or several amino acids giving them lower scores.

Food	Fiber (g)
Beans (½ cup)	6–10
Apple/Pear (1 medium)	5
Wheat cereal (1 cup)	5–7
Popcorn (1 cup)	4
Banana (1 medium)	3
Lentil soup (1 cup)	8
Wheat bread (1 slice)	3

Before you begin hyperventilating and thinking that you are going to be shopping for specific amino acids at the grocery store, rest assured that is not the case. I mention the specifics of protein biochemistry simply to underscore the idea that not all protein-containing foods provide the same quality protein. Furthermore, this concept provides the perfect platform to begin the discussion of variety and moderation. By choosing a variety of protein sources in your family's diet, you are more likely to ensure that every amino acid is obtained in adequate amounts throughout the day.

Protein-containing foods should be part of every meal or snack that you and your family choose. Protein takes a bit longer to digest than carbohydrates, thus offering a lingering feeling of satiety when included in a meal or snack. We tend to do an okay job of including protein at meal time, however very few of us choose lean protein at snack time. One terrific goal when shopping for proteins is to choose portable, kid-friendly protein sources that are easily combined with

---

Calculating Your Ideal Body Weight (IBW)

Women: Add 100 pounds for your first 5 feet plus an additional 5 pounds for each inch over 5 feet. Example: A woman who is 5' 4" would add 100 + (5 x 4") = 120 pounds.

Men: Add 106 pounds for your first 5 feet plus an additional 6 pounds for each inch over 5 feet. Example: A man who is 5'11" would add 106 + (6 x 11") = 172 pounds.

To convert weight from pounds to kilograms, divide pounds by 2.2. 150 pounds = 150/2.2 = 54.54 kg.

Daily Protein Needs at Any Age	
Age	**Protein (g/kg of IBW)**
0–6 months	2.2
6 months–1year	1.6
1–3	1.2
4–6	1.1
7–10	1.0
11–14 boy	1.0
11–14 girl	1.0
15–18 boy	0.9
15–18 girl	0.85
Adults	0.8–1.2

fiber-full carbohydrates to make a great on-the-go snack. Some easy examples are low-fat string cheese and berries, an apple with peanut butter, cottage cheese and peaches, turkey slices and pears, yogurt and whole grain cereal, to name just a few.

How much protein do you need? For children, protein needs range from 2 g/kg ideal body weight all the way up to the adult requirements that range from 0.8 to 1.2 g/kg of ideal body weight. For a 150 pound woman, those numbers translate into a daily protein requirement of 55 grams or about 8 ounces. For a 175 pound man, the daily protein needs are around 80 grams or 11.5 ounces.

You don't have to look far to find protein powders and supplements that offer nearly half of the average total daily protein requirement in one small serving. Unless you are an Olympic body builder, choosing such supplements is often un-necessary and potentially harmful if used over a long period of time. Ideally, your protein needs would be met by including high-quality protein in moderate serving sizes each time you eat throughout the day.

There are certain instances where having too much protein in the diet can be harmful. For people with kidney disease, there is often a restriction on how much protein to include each day, as protein is filtered by the kidney and too much can be taxing. If you have any type of

Food	Protein (g)
1 egg	7
3 oz. chicken	21
1 Greek yogurt	12
1 cup kidney beans	13
3 oz. salmon	21
1 veggie burger	10
1 oz. tofu	4.5
1 oz. cheese	7
1 Clif Builder's bar	21

kidney issue, it is a good idea to consult with your physician before determining how much protein to include in your diet each day.

Fats

Having grown up in the '80s and '90s, I am part of the "fat-free generation." A product only needed to be labeled fat free in the '90s, and it automatically shot to the top of the health food list. During that period, companies produced a plethora of products that were "fat free," yet high in sugar. It was the belief at the time that if we did not eat fat, we would not get fat. However, quite the opposite reaction occurred. The rate of obesity from the early '80s to today has nearly doubled. In 1980, 5 percent of men and 8 percent of women were obese in the United States, compared to 10 percent of men and 14 percent of women in 2008.

It is amazing how much things have changed since then. Now, in order to be healthy, you have to include fat in your diet. Where were all the biochemists in 1993? I could have skipped the 10 pounds I gained my freshman year in college on sugary (fat-free) cereal and licorice (also brilliantly fat free). Nevertheless, now we know how our body metabolizes fats and how to include heart-healthy fats in our diet in moderation to help us stay satisfied and achieve improved health.

Fats are found in both animal- and plant-based foods. The variation in their chemical structure identifies them as either being saturated, monounsaturated, or polyunsaturated. Familiar sources of saturated fat include butter, fatty meat, high-fat dairy, and coconut and palm oils. Polyunsaturated fats are found in certain vegetable oils, such as sunflower, corn, and safflower, as well as omega-3 fats found in fish and flaxseed. The most heart-healthy type of fat is monounsaturated. This group includes olive oil, canola oil, nuts, and avocado. All three types of fats provide essential fatty acids that play many chemical and structural roles within our bodies.

The types of fats we include in our diet can have a measurable impact on our cardiovascular health. Intake of saturated fat is associated with an increased risk for cardiovascular disease because it raises our total cholesterol. Furthermore, saturated fats tend to be sticky, causing plaque production and clogged arteries. Conversely, heart-healthy fats, such as some polyunsaturated fats and monounsaturated fats, can actually improve the cholesterol profile by raising the HDL (good cholesterol) without raising our total cholesterol. The ratio of total cholesterol to HDL cholesterol is a predictor of heart disease risk; therefore, the higher the HDL the better.

Grocery shopping for healthy fats should be focused on selecting monounsaturated and polyunsaturated fats that can be used in small servings throughout the day. A few good examples are peanut butter, almonds, tuna, salmon, olive oil, and avocado.

The Nitty-Gritty: Food at the Micronutrient Level

Although you are well on your way to earning your honorary degree in food science, we cannot grant you your cap and gown without touching on the importance of micronutrients in our diets. Micronutrients include vitamins and minerals, as well as other chemicals, that are naturally part of a food's structure and bestow health benefits upon our bodies. The U.S. government helps us understand these micronutrients by creating Recommended Daily Intake (RDI) guidelines for several key nutrients, including vitamins A, B, C, and D, as well as calcium, iron, potassium, zinc, and sodium. The percent daily values (%DV) are listed on every food label in the market. They indicate what percentage of the nutrient that particular food provides when following a 2,000 calorie/day diet.

I recognize that this can be really confusing! How many of us actually know to the calorie what our total caloric intake is each day? Are we expected to add up our daily percentages of each nutrient throughout the day to ensure our vitamin and mineral intakes are adequate? No, of course not. However, reading labels and comparing nutrient density in some of your favorite foods can be a guide toward better health.

Vitamins are essential nutrients to the human body. They are only required in small quantities, setting them apart from the larger macronutrient groupings we have already discussed. Vitamins function within our bodies in many ways. They are essentially the "worker bees" within our hive; directing traffic, creating pathways, and assisting others. Vitamins can be divided into two categories—water-soluble and fat-soluble. Water-soluble vitamins, including B-vitamins and vitamin C, are not stored in our bodies to any great extent. Because they are easily dissolved in water, excess water-soluble vitamins are excreted in our urine. Therefore, it is important to ensure adequate intakes of these vitamins each day.

Fat-soluble vitamins, which include vitamins A, D, E, and K, are absorbed and stored differently by our bodies. It is therefore more likely that we could accumulate excess fat-soluble vitamins in our bodies, leading to potential complications.

Commonly, people eating a well-balanced diet do not need any additional vitamin or mineral supplements. However, if you do decide to add a vitamin/mineral supplement to your diet, it is important to pay attention to the RDI percentage on the nutrition label. You never need a multivitamin that provides 5,000 percent of the RDI of a nutrient. Foods and supplements are intended to contribute to your total needs, not to surpass them by 4,900 percent. A good rule of thumb is to choose foods and supplements with RDI percentages that are under 100 percent. This way, when the day is over, all of your good choices combined together meet your daily needs.

The easiest way to ensure that you and your family are receiving adequate vitamin intake on a regular basis is to focus on color, servings, and variety. Fruits and vegetables retain certain colors based on the types of vitamins and minerals they contain. Typically, the deeper the color, the more nutrient-dense a fruit or vegetable may be. By choosing a variety of colors of fruits and vegetables throughout the day and week, you will help to ensure that the required vitamins and minerals are being received. This can be a fun way for kids to think about being healthy as well. Encourage them to "eat the rainbow" when it comes to produce.

It is recommended that most adults consume roughly two cups of fruit and two and a half cups of vegetables each day. Since most of us eat about 5 times during the day (3 meals and 2 snacks), each time we eat there should be a serving of fruit and/or a vegetable as part of the meal to ensure that we are meeting our micronutrient needs.

Minerals, including calcium, sodium, potassium, phosphorus, chlorine, sulfur, iron, zinc, and magnesium, are essential to the human body and function as both structural components and electrolytes within our body. Our bones would not grow and our muscles would not contract without them.

Minerals are found throughout our food supply and there is a great deal of nutritional propaganda focused on their consumption. Get enough calcium, decrease your sodium intake, seek out potassium-containing foods, supplement zinc—the list goes on and on. Choosing a diet primarily comprised of whole foods, limiting canned and processed items, is likely to ensure safe mineral consumption.

Calcium is one of the key minerals that is often lacking in the American diet. For example, teenagers' calcium needs are roughly 1,300 mg per day. That equates to about 5 servings of a calcium-containing food a day. In my 14 years of practice, I have yet to meet a teen that ingests that much healthy dairy each day. This is an example of a great opportunity to supplement the diet with a calcium supplement. One 500 mg calcium supplement added to the diet each day means that this teen now only needs 3 servings of a calcium-containing food to meet his or her needs. Specific nutrient needs, including calcium, will be discussed when we identify great sources for these key nutrients throughout the book.

If shopping for an athlete is on your agenda, electrolytes are likely a buzzword in your home. Most athletes do not realize that they can replenish the electrolytes they lose from sweat by eating a good meal. The need for specific electrolyte replacement is truly limited to the exerciser who is putting in more than 60 minutes of intense physical activity at a time. Our bodies are extremely efficient at maintaining a homeostasis at the cellular level in the average person on an average day. Yes, that means your little leaguer doesn't need a 60-ounce bottle of Gatorade after running the bases.

Cheers to Your Good Health!

I know it is rare to clink your water glasses, but there is truly no greater way to toast to your good health. For many, staying hydrated proves to be the exclamation point at the end of the perfect nutrition sentence. Hydration has the power to help curb cravings, speed metabolism, stave off hunger, energize, improve performance, and heighten awareness. Drinking at least eight 8-ounce glasses of water each day will help to ensure that you maintain a proper hydration status all of the time.

While needs vary in some populations (pregnancy, elderly, small children, athletes, cardiac, and kidney patients), most average teens and adults require that 64 ounces of water (1,920 ml). For most people, this equates to roughly one half glass every hour you are awake. Hydration needs for the athlete or avid exerciser are elevated as we lose a great deal of water in our sweat. Replace water loss from exercise with one extra glass for every half-hour you sweat. The average adult who works out for an hour a day will now need ten 8-ounce glasses each day.

Seek out a great water bottle. Having a water bottle that you enjoy drinking from can be the secret to success in the hydration department. Calculate how many times you need to refill that specific bottle each day to meet your needs and you are all set.

Congratulations! You have just finished the layperson's

equivalent of the extremely detailed organic and biochemistry classes that I had to complete in undergraduate school. This information will provide the basis for your further education on how to combine key nutrients to create healthy meals and snacks for any occasion. It will also allow you to delve deeper into your family's connection to food and to strategize for any situation that involves a meal or snack, which is pretty much every situation when you have kids! The choice to feed your family in a positive and mindful way is just as multidimensional in its approach as it is in the level of reward that your family will reap. Hang on and enjoy the ride to nutritional serenity.

Method to
the Madness

When I meet with clients, I have one primary goal. Through education and counseling, my clients will develop a healthy and peaceful relationship with food and their bodies. This goal is the same whether the client is 7 or 70, whether they are overweight or underweight. In order to reach this objective, many distractions, both physical and psychological, must be eliminated from my clients' lives to allow for the peace and clarity to set in. The three main things that I focus my counseling on are controlling insulin production, developing a game plan, and becoming a mindful eater. When these three concepts are in place, my clients claim that they have never felt more in control and free when it comes their diet. By understanding these concepts, trips to the grocery store and meal time preparation also become more peaceful and productive.

Maintaining a healthy weight through a balanced diet will

impact every single aspect of your life. Proper nutrition and a healthy weight will encourage you to be more active. Similarly, it will reduce your risk for a number of chronic diseases, reduce medical costs, improve performance, increase productivity, and raise self-esteem. When you stop and think about it, what you made for dinner has such a wide scope of impact. If you are a parent, you will certainly find that the influence of good nutrition is felt in every aspect of your parenting as well.

The key to maintaining a healthy weight over the course of our lifetime is to control our body's production of insulin. The rapid increase in the number of cases of type 2 diabetes in the United States over the course of the last two decades indicates that, as a population, we do a very poor job of curbing the body's insulin production. In fact, the National Health and Nutrition Examination Survey showed that the percentage of teenagers testing positive for diabetes and pre-diabetes had nearly tripled to 23 percent in 2007–2008 from 9 percent in 1999–2000. This large jump in diabetes rates has everything to do with the poor quality of our diets and the inadequacy of our level of physical activity on a given day. But this is an avoidable trend.

Insulin production is very simply controlled by following three main rules:

1. **Choose foods in combination.** The foods that always need to be present in a meal or a snack are fiber-full carbohydrates and lean protein. A couple of times a day, we will also add in healthy fats. I explain this concept

to kids by using the best friend analogy. I tell my clients that fiber-full carbohydrates and lean proteins are best friends. They like to be together at every meal and snack, no matter what. Most kids have a best friend with whom they want to do everything, making this an easy concept to understand.

2. **Eat often.** By choosing a meal or a snack every 3–4 hours, we ensure that our blood sugar levels stay in a moderate zone. This prevents cravings and the uninhibited or mindless eating that often takes place after long periods without food. Maintaining a steady blood sugar throughout the day is crucial for long-term success.

3. **Exercise regularly.** Regular exercise is a necessary piece of the health puzzle. Our bodies were meant to participate in physical activity. As an adult, there are limitless options for getting fit. If you are also a parent, there is perhaps no greater lesson to teach your children than the importance of regular physical activity. Be a role model to your family and friends by setting aside time each day for exercise. For those of you who are parents, choose family friendly activities that challenge and empower yourself and your children. Visit www.active.com to locate 1-mile and 5-kilometer races. Purchase hula hoops and jump ropes for an inexpensive and fun way to increase your heart rate. Go for bike rides, walks, and jogs together. Play your Wii Fit together. Purchase a kickboxing DVD that the whole family will enjoy.

These three concepts seem obvious when you read them. Unfortunately, they are very seldom followed by many individuals. The quality of your diet is self-promoting, meaning that when you eat well it spurs more good choices throughout the day. Similarly, a poor choice at some point during the day often leads to more poor choices as the day and week go on. This is because an erratic blood sugar leads to cravings for low-quality nutrition. One handful of a fiber-less carbohydrate will create the "need" for more of that type of food throughout the day. This is the feeling of "just needing something sweet or salty" with which we are all familiar.

If you are able to follow the rules of eating often and eating in combination, cravings begin to disappear. When the cravings are few and far between, the common sense and nutrition knowledge you have gained come into focus. Each time you choose a meal or a snack, you are thinking with your head and not your tummy. You are also less likely to give in to peer pressure when it comes to food. We often choose foods because of what our friends or coworkers are eating. For parents, educating your kids on how and why you choose certain foods will allow them to be able to make a good choice anywhere, even if you are not there to guide.

Cravings are eliminated when our diets are composed of fiber-full carbohydrates, lean proteins, healthy fats, and plenty of hydration. Our bodies reward us for taking care of them by making us feel good. When we eat this way 90 percent of the time, our bodies allow us the flexibility of enjoying treats in moderation throughout the week or month.

I would never advocate for a world where birthday cake wasn't allowed! And I would also never advocate for a world where Monday was ice cream night, Tuesday was slushy day, Wednesday was cookies at Grandma's, Thursday was frozen coffee drink with whipped cream and caramel day, and Friday was baking night. We are all being exposed to treats multiple times a day, and our nutrition parameters are being challenged at every turn. This makes eating well during that 90 percent of the week even that much more important.

Plan for Perfection

We plan for everything. We stay up late prepping for meetings at work, do the laundry so the baseball uniform is clean from Monday to Wednesday, buy construction paper so the school project can be completed, pay bills, plan for vacations, shop for clothes, and save for college. So how come most of us don't plan for our diets?

In my private practice, I find that the main reason most people walk aimlessly through the food world is that they simply do not know where to begin. But you do not have that excuse any longer. You are more than knowledgeable when it comes to what makes a healthy meal or snack. You would not leave your house in the morning without your briefcase or smartphone, and you should not leave for work or send your kids to school or a sporting event without the proper nutrition either. Planning for any situation is more than half the battle when it comes to food.

The ice pack is perhaps the most underrated item in the

kitchen. I love the soft flexible ones. They usually only cost about two dollars and are bendable, allowing them to fit into any bag or even wrap around a carton of yogurt or a sandwich. There are very few nutritious items that do not need to be kept cold, so have plenty of ice packs around in order to pack something great for every member of the family.

Along those same lines, having great lunch bags and snack bags is a must. There are a number of eco-friendly bags on the market now that are dishwasher-safe, making them easy to use each day. Teenagers seem to have the most difficult time packing the reusable bag. I've been told it is simply not cool to have a lunch bag. In that case, a ziplock plastic bag full of ice can act as a disposable ice pack and a brown paper bag can carry the meal or snack to school or work. Simply put, there is no excuse for being unprepared.

Create a game plan for any situation. If you are leaving your house in the morning and will not return until the evening, you have to have water and snacks with you, even if you plan to have a lunch away from home. You know this because you have to eat every 3 to 4 hours, and that those meals and snacks must have fiber-full carbohydrates and lean protein in them. These are not things that are typically found in a vending machine. Packing a bag with a serving of fruit and a serving of vegetables is a great place to start. Add in a light string cheese or ounce of almonds (about 15), a single serving of hummus, or an ounce of whole grain cereal and you are well on your way. Your snack might consist of a healthy sandwich (whole grain bread or wrap with a few slices of turkey) or a small cottage cheese with slices of pineapple. You can already tell that these options sound more filling than a candy bar or bag of pretzels and you will feel more healthful when you eat better.

The student athlete has a unique scenario when it comes to snacking. They often go to the gym or have sports directly following school and have to change and eat something quickly before starting. They also have been away from home for more than 7 hours in many instances, making anything that needs to remain refrigerated no longer cold even with an ice pack. This is a perfect place to introduce nutrition or protein bars. While I would not advocate that bars replace every meal or snack, there is a tremendous benefit to using them in certain situations and this is certainly one of them. Some bars are excellent in that they combine the key nutrients (fiber-full carbs, lean protein, and healthy fat) so that they are a perfect meal or snack all on their own. (We will explore nutrition bars when we go through the aisles of the grocery store in coming chapters.)

Long work days and travel days pose similar challenges. If you have access to a fridge at your office, use it! Bring in a shopping bag full of healthy options at the beginning of the week so you always have good choices from which to choose. For whatever reason, people have turned the workplace into a nutrition minefield. Everyone is guilty of bringing their leftover cakes and cookies to the office and leaving them in the break room. The access to low-quality nutrition coupled with the often stressful environment at the office tends to equate to poor food choices. If you have made the effort to bring in fruits, veggies, hard-boiled eggs, light cheese, yogurt, turkey slices, etc., you are likely to choose those things in lieu of the candy or cake.

If your work takes you away from the office and a fridge is not an option, have no fear—sound nutrition is still possible. Many of us carry smartphones in our purses and pockets, which can be a tremendous help when it comes to making good food choices. There are several free apps that give you access to the nutritional value of the menu options at chain restaurants. Having such an app on your phone could allow you to stop in a Subway for a 6" turkey sub on whole wheat or choose a healthy egg white wrap at a Starbucks. If you spend a great deal of time in your car, consider purchasing a cooler for the car that plugs into the lighter. This would allow you the freedom to pack all sorts of healthy options when you are on the go all day.

Mindful Eating

When you choose the right foods to keep in your house, and then go the extra step of bringing them with you each day to work or school, you begin to create a very peaceful way of living. Sure, there is a great deal of work that goes into always having fresh produce and a stocked pantry, but it is just as much work to shop for unhealthy foods as it is to shop for healthy ones. This newfound level of serenity when it comes to eating allows you to be more present or aware each time you make a choice about food. Entering into a meal or snack time with a steady blood sugar feels different than coming to the dinner table with a low blood sugar. Now you are in control of the food instead of feeling as though the food is in control of you.

You are now able to embrace the concept of "mindful eating." Mindful eating has been shown in numerous studies not only to decrease your total caloric intake, but also to improve metabolism and overall well-being. Mindful eating begins before the food hits your mouth. I teach the concept of self-reflection when it comes to making choices. This means that you have to talk to yourself a bit before you eat something. It is often helpful to come up with three questions that you ask yourself before you eat. My questions are:

1. Am I really hungry?
2. Will I be happy I ate this food in two hours?
3. Is there something else I could choose that would be better for my body and mind at this moment?

If the answers to the questions all check out, then proceed and enjoy. If the answer to one of those questions is no, then it is time to alter your choice to one that will make you feel good. Just as I said at the beginning of this chapter, the quality of your diet is self-promoting. If you feel good about your choices, you are likely to continue to make great choices throughout the day. If you make a choice that leaves you feeling regretful, you are likely to take less pride in yourself the rest of the day, which undoubtedly will result in even more poor choices.

After you have decided on the type of food you are going

to eat, it is important to eat it in a mindful way as well. Look at the food, smell it, think about it. Take your time while eating. Enjoy one bite and place your fork back on the table. Turn off the television, hang up the phone, and put the newspaper away. When we eat while we are doing other things, we tend not to realize how much we are eating. When we focus on the food in front of us, we eat less. We notice that our bodies are being satisfied sooner. The old adage that "the calories you consume while standing in front of the refrigerator do not count" unfortunately is not true.

It is an eye-opening exercise to document everything you eat on a given day. You will be surprised by the number of calories you consume when you are not eating a planned meal or snack. The crusts off your child's peanut butter and jelly sandwich, a spoonful of mac-n-cheese, two fries, a few M&M's at the office—those calories add up! Practice being mindful one day at a time.

Teach your children to slow down when they eat as well. Talk to them about how you prepared the food and from where the food came. Plant a garden to enhance your appreciation for the food you eat each day. Each and every one of these processes will contribute to an overall heightened awareness of the food choices you and your family make.

The mastery of the principles of insulin control, strategy development, and mindful eating are required prerequisites for supermarket serenity. You should notice a sense of control and purpose begin to emerge. This refreshing sensation will help to drive you each and every day. It will grant you the clarity you need to teach your family and serve as a role model. It will give you the freedom to grocery shop with confidence and resolve.

Planning for Perfection at the Market

In order to be an effective grocery shopper you need to know and understand what you are looking for in each product. Each food you pick up in the market is subject to a different litmus test of health. For example, when shopping for cereals, we would pay special attention to grams of sugar and fiber, as cereals are a carbohydrate-based food, and carbohydrates contribute both sugar and fiber to our diets. When shopping for ground beef we wouldn't look at either of those things. Rather we would focus on total fat, protein, and calories to determine if we were making a good choice. This is because ground beef is a protein and protein foods contribute fat, protein, and calories to our diet. Lastly, when grabbing a bottle of cooking oil, the first place my eye would look would be to the types of fat that it provides, as oil is a fat and thus contributes fat to our diet. Understanding which nutrients our foods provide to us will be a helpful guide as you determine which choices are best for you and your family.

Reading a Food Label

The Nutrition Facts panel provides information on the nutritional composition of each food we purchase in the market with the exception of fresh produce, meat, and poultry. In 1990, the Nutrition Labeling and Education Act (NLEA) was introduced as law. The law mandated that food companies begin using the new food label on packaged foods starting May 8, 1994. This food label is now printed on over 6.5 million food items throughout the world. Certain requirements exist for the minimum amount of nutrition information that must appear on each food label. This list includes serving size, calories per serving, calories from fat, total fat, saturated fat, trans fat, cholesterol, sodium, total carbohydrates, dietary fiber, protein, vitamin A, vitamin C, calcium, and iron.

There is a certain art to reading labels. After you read enough of them, you begin to get the hang of it and you'll be able to do it very quickly. The first stop when reading labels should always be serving size. Too often, food manufacturers try to fool consumers by offering more than one serving in a seemingly small package. This obviously makes the Nutrition Facts panel look a lot more nutrition-friendly, when in fact it is not. The Nutrition Facts panel (Fig. 1) shows that there are 4 servings of the food in this package. If you were to choose something like this and see that there are supposed to be 4 servings in the package, yet you know that this package will clearly only provide 2 servings, then you must multiply all of the nutrition information by two in order to see what it will really provide to you or someone for whom you are cooking.

Once you have determined that the serving size is reasonable, it is time to look at total calories. Whether you are shopping for cereal, snacks, or soup, the total calories that a food provides is an excellent checkpoint to see if the food fits within your nutritional parameters. While each of us needs a different number of total calories to maintain a healthy weight,

Nutrition Facts

Serving Size 1/2 cup (115g)
Servings Per Container About 4

Amount Per Serving

Calories 250	Calories from Fat 130

	% Daily Value*
Total Fat 14g	**22%**
Saturated Fat 9g	**45%**
Cholesterol 55mg	**18%**
Sodium 75mg	**3%**
Total Carbohydrate 26g	**9%**
Dietary Fiber 0g	**0%**
Sugars 26g	
Protein 4g	

Vitamin A 10%	Vitamin C 0%
Calcium 10%	Iron 0%

* Percent Daily Values are based on a 2,000 calorie diet.

Figure 1. A Nutrition Facts Panel

certain commonsense guidelines can be applied to the majority of the population. Most adults and teens should consume somewhere between 1,500 and 2,500 calories per day. That means that, if you eat three meals and two snacks, any given snack should likely be around 200 calories and any meal should hover somewhere around 500 calories. Let's say that you pick up a box of frozen pizza snacks. Each serving may have around 250 calories depending on the flavor. That number of total calories may be an automatic "no thank you," as you know that it exceeds the calories you had hoped to consume in your snack. On the other hand, if you pick up a seemingly healthy frozen dinner and find the total calories to be around 400, you should keep reading as the total calories fall within an acceptable range for a meal.

Once the serving size and total calories have checked out, the label reading becomes a bit more specific. Remembering a few key rules can make this process easier.

1. When purchasing carbohydrate foods (breads, cereals, pastas, rice, crackers, snacks, cookies, granola bars, chips), it is important to always look for grams of fiber and grams of sugar.

   • Ideally, most of the carbohydrates you purchase will contain dietary fiber. A good amount of dietary fiber is more than 3 grams per serving.

   • Unfortunately, many carbohydrate-based foods tend to be high in sugar. Unless you are choosing a food with natural sugar present, such as fruit, milk, or yogurt, the threshold of less than 10 grams of sugar per serving is a good one to follow.

2. When purchasing protein-containing foods (cheese milk, yogurt, meats, poultry, fish, eggs), it is important to look at grams of protein and grams of fat.

   • Most protein-containing foods will contain some fat, so we are not necessarily looking for zero grams. However, you can use the total grams of fat to help you decide between two similar products. For example, when shopping for cheese, you will notice that the reduced-fat varieties have roughly half the fat as the full-fat vareties, yet they contain the same number of grams of protein. Hopefully, this will motivate you to make the healthier choice and choose the low-fat cheese.

- The amount of protein in protein-based foods tends not to differ dramatically between most similar products. One ounce of cheese will always have the same amount of protein, whether it is reduced-fat or not. When you read a label for protein, you are really looking to see if that particular item provides an adequate amount of protein for its intended purpose. This is easily illustrated by using the frozen entrée example. If you are purchasing a frozen entrée that you intend for dinner, but you read the label and there are only 12 grams of protein, you may want to think again. Most meals should provide at least 14 to 21 grams of protein or the equivalent of 3 ounces of meat or poultry in order to be satisfying for most adults. At snack time, the goal would be to have at least 7 grams of protein, or the equivalent of 1 ounce of protein.

3. Lastly, when choosing primarily fat-based foods like oils, nuts, and avocados, your objective is to seek out the healthiest blends of fats. Lower numbers of grams of saturated fats and trans fats are ideal, as are higher numbers of monounsaturated fats. The Nutrition Facts panel on a package of heart-healthy almonds shows that there are 12 grams of fat per 200 calorie serving, but only 0.5 g of those 12 grams is saturated fat, which makes almonds a great choice.

Several other key nutrients are listed on the Nutrition Facts panel. Total cholesterol is listed in mg (milligrams). Cholesterol will only be found in animal-based products, so we would not expect there to be any cholesterol in a can of beans or an apple. The American Heart Association recommends that all Americans limit total cholesterol intake to less than 300 mg per day. If you already have been identified as having high cholesterol, then your total daily intake should be less than 200 mg. An 8-ounce steak has about 200 mg, and one egg yolk has 213 mg, just to put those numbers in perspective. Typically, by choosing a healthy diet in moderation we are able to keep blood cholesterol levels in a healthy range.

Checking food labels for sodium can be an eye-opening experience. Sodium is a mineral that has the potential to negatively impact our blood pressure when present in high concentrations in our diet. Most well-hydrated children and adults who have no kidney issues can tolerate higher sodium intakes. Americans, on average, consume 8,000–10,000 mg of sodium a day. The American Heart Association guidelines recommend less than 2,000 mg per day. This discrepancy is largely due to our dependence on processed, canned, and boxed foods, which use sodium as a flavor enhancer and preservative. A higher-sodium food choice here or there is likely not a problem for the average consumer. However, if you find that you rely heavily on processed foods, it may be time to make a shift. A serving of canned soup can have upwards of 1,000 mg of sodium, as does one pickle or two ounces of salami. Choose more fresh, whole foods to help reduce your regular sodium intake.

Without adequate potassium in our diets, our heart, lungs, and muscles would not work properly. In fact, the DASH (Dietary Approaches to Stop Hypertension) diet illustrates how a diet that is high in potassium can help to lower high blood pressure and risk for heart disease. Potassium is listed on every food label in mg (milligrams.) Choosing plenty of fruits, vegetables, and beans will help to ensure that there is adequate potassium intake throughout the day. Certain individuals who are on specific medications, such as diuretics, or those with kidney disease should consult their physician to determine a safe level of potassium intake.

Vitamins A and C, as well as calcium and iron, are the last required nutrients to be listed on the Nutrition Facts panel. These micronutrients are listed with the Percent Daily Values they provide based on a 2,000 calorie diet. These percentages are useful in determining "good sources" for these particular nutrients. The Nutrition Facts panel on a can of artichoke hearts shows that one serving provides greater than 100 percent of your daily vitamin C needs. In general, glancing at these numbers can be educational and interesting, yet they are not likely to determine whether you purchase a specific product or not.

What Is Really in There?

Just below the Nutrition Facts panel sits the ingredient list. This complete listing of both natural and artificial ingredients gives greater insight into the food you are considering. Some health professionals would say it is simply a good rule of thumb to avoid any food whose ingredients you cannot pronounce. If you follow this rule, however, you would likely eliminate about 90 percent of the foods sold in most conventional grocery stores around the country. More practical advice may be to learn about some common food additives, their safety profile and functional purpose, and then decide for yourself which ones deserve a place on your pantry shelf.

Ingredient lists are conveniently listed in order of their concentration within a product. This means that if sugar is the first ingredient on a list, it is the ingredient that, by weight, is in the highest concentration. Whether your focus in the grocery store is weight loss or general health, reviewing the ingredient lists of the common foods you purchase is a proactive way of becoming a more informed shopper.

If you pick up a box, bag, or jar in the market, chances are there will be some sort of food additives listed in the ingredient list. There are hundreds of food additives in our current food supply. Simply type the words "food additive" into your computer's search engine and you will have enough reading material for the next decade. Seven common food additives seem to have garnered the most attention, albeit mostly negative. This list includes food colorings, high fructose corn syrup, aspartame, MSG (monosodium gluta-mate), sodium benzoate, sodium nitrate, and trans fats. If you intend to be a grocery genius, the use, purpose, and safety of these additives should be part of your vocabulary.

There are large differences between individual reactions to

ingredients. Much of this portion of your nutrition education may need to be more personalized based on your own observational evidence. Remember, your neighbor may be extremely sensitive to a particular food additive, while the same ingredient elicits no response by your body. If you notice that after eating certain foods, you develop symptoms, take note of which additives or preservatives are listed on the label. This is the single best way to determine your own guidelines.

Artificial Colorings

As famous dietitian quotes go, "Eat the rainbow" is up there on the list. The concept behind eating lots of different colored fruits and vegetables is that produce gets its deep colors from the types of vitamins and minerals it contains. Therefore, by choosing a variety of colored fruits and vegetables you get a variety of nutrients in your diet. Unfortunately, food manufacturers use a lot of artificial colorings to make their products more appealing. While many colorings have been removed from our food supply over the years because of their known carcinogenic effect, several remain in regular use and pose a potential risk. Examples include:

1. Yellow #5, which has been linked to hyperactivity.
2. Red #3, which caused thyroid tumors in rats in a 1983 study.
3. Red #40, which is the most widely used food coloring, can cause allergic reactions in sensitive individuals.
4. Blue #2 showed some evidence of brain cancer pro-

motion in rodents, yet the FDA's position is that there is "reasonable certainty of no harm."

Sweeteners

High fructose corn syrup (HFCS) has been blamed for everything from the obesity epidemic to the poor economy. (Well, maybe not that, but I'm sure there is some claim to that effect!) This man-made ingredient contains the same combination of fructose and glucose that cane sugar does, just in slightly different proportions. There has been great discussion that the combination of these two sugars in high fructose corn syrup is more likely to create weight gain and increase our risk for type 2 diabetes as compared to table sugar. Most of this evidence is anecdotal at best, as there is no single study that shows that excess HFCS consumption in humans leads to more weight gain than excess cane sugar consumption. The reality is that too much consumption of any sugar is not healthy for anyone. When reading labels, it would be advised to commonly choose foods that have minimal added sugar.

I am sure you have heard that aspartame (aka NutraSweet or Equal) causes cancer, brain tumors, headaches, depression, attention deficit disorder, etc. The truth is that aspartame, an artificial sweetener commonly used in diet soft drinks and other low-calorie foods such as yogurts and puddings, is probably one of the most studied ingredients in our food supply. There have been more than 25 published studies over the last two decades that have shown no correlation between aspartame intake and increased incidence of leukemia, lymphoma, or brain tumors. Even the National Cancer Institute, which looked at a meta-analysis of 500,000 adults, showed no correlation between aspartame consumption and cancer risk.

That being said, I always think common sense is required when it comes to food. Would I choose to include multiple foods each day in my diet that were filled with artificial sweeteners? Probably not. However, there are certain foods like an occasional diet soda or a light yogurt that fit well within a calorie-controlled diet that I would consider.

For those of you shopping for children, I would take special precaution when it comes to artificial sweeteners and err on the side of caution. In my private practice, the only artificially sweetened foods I tend to recommend for kids are yogurts. In my clinical mind, the benefits of choosing a high-calcium, high-protein food such as yogurt for part of a meal or a snack far outweigh the perceived risk of the minimal amount of artificial sweetener that it contains.

Other sweeteners that are commonly found in foods include sucralose (Splenda), Rebiana (stevia extract, Truvia), Neotame, acesulfame potassium (Ace-K), and saccharin. These sweeteners are often used in conjunction with one another to create the perfect sweetness without an aftertaste. Clinical studies on sucralose have made this artificial sweetener one that I feel comfortable recommending for clients to enjoy occasionally. Newer additives such as Rebiana have not been around long enough to gather longitudinal evidence.

Using common sense and limiting artificially sweetened products is likely best.

Flavor Enhancers

Monosodium glutamate (MSG) is a flavor enhancer most famously known as an additive in Chinese food. MSG is often used in soups, salad dressings, and frozen meals, yet many people are very sensitive to its presence. Glutamate is an amino acid that is naturally present in foods, such as parmesan cheese and tomatoes, and it can even be found in other natural flavors. If you are one of the people who develop symptoms such as nausea and headache from consuming foods with MSG, be sure to avoid such items by reading your labels carefully.

The sodium twins, sodium benzoate and sodium nitrate, are added to foods as preservatives and flavoring. Sodium benzoate is a naturally occurring compound, yet when it is used in acidic beverages that contain vitamin C, an unfortunate chemical reaction takes place producing benzene, a known carcinogen. Several beverage companies were actually sued in 2006, forcing them to modify the use of this additive.

Would you buy a gray hot dog? Of course not, and that is why food producers add sodium nitrite and sodium nitrate to processed and cured meats. The risk associated with overconsumption of these additives is that nitrite can lead to the production of the carcinogen nitrosamine. This conversion is greatly hindered by the addition of ascorbic acid, yet there is still a risk associated with choosing foods regularly that contain such additives. This is where common sense checks back into the game. Bacon, ham, and hot dogs should not be major components of your daily diet. You probably knew that before you began reading this book, yet a little dose of reality is always important. Choosing all foods in moderation is the mantra, and it is certainly true with processed meats.

Added Fats

Trans fats, often seen labeled as "partially hydrogenated vegetable oil," have taken a roller coaster ride over the past few decades. Initially touted as a healthier alternative to the saturated fat found in butter and shortening, trans fats are now known to be more dangerous than the saturated fats they were intended to replace. In 2004, the FDA urged food manufacturers to limit the use of this additive, and in 2006, trans fat was mandated to be identified on food labels. Most of the large packaged-food producers have changed their formulations to be "trans-fat free," and many chain restaurants have jumped on the band wagon as well. In fact, consumption of trans fat dropped 50 percent over the past decade. It is advised that consumption of trans fats should be limited to less than 2 grams per day.

While the above list is obviously not an exhaustive one, it sheds light on some of the things that I, as a dietitian, consider when making a recommendation to include or limit a specific food or additive. Using the concept of moderation is obviously critical when it comes to this conversation.

There is always research being conducted on food and its ingredients, so the facts we know to be true today regarding a certain additive can change overnight with new findings. By choosing mostly whole foods and other foods in moderation, I think that food can be nourishing and not menacing.

To Organic or Not to Organic, That Is the Question

The United States Department of Agriculture's National Organic Program (NOP) has been legislating the production and labeling of organic foods since 2002. The laws overseen by the NOP guarantee that foods sold and labeled as organic are held to the highest of organic standards. The NOP defines organic as follows:

Organic food is produced by farmers who emphasize the use of renewable resources and the conservation of soil and water to enhance environmental quality for future generations. Organic meat, poultry, eggs, and dairy products come from animals that are given no antibiotics or growth hormones. Organic food is produced without using most conventional pesticides; fertilizers made with synthetic ingredients or sewage sludge; bioengineering; or ionizing radiation. Before a product can be labeled "organic," a Government-approved certifier inspects the farm where the food is grown to make sure the farmer is following all the rules necessary to meet USDA organic standards. Companies that handle or process organic food before it gets to your local supermarket or restaurant must be certified, too.

When reading labels, you may notice that the "organicity"

The Dirty Dozen
Apples
Celery
Strawberries
Peaches
Spinach
Nectarines (imported)
Grapes (imported, and raisins, too!)
Sweet peppers
Potatoes (sweet potatoes have fewer pesticides)
Blueberries
Lettuce
Kale and collard greens

of a certain product is labeled in many different ways. Claims including "100 percent organic" may appear on labels indicating that all of the ingredients used, with the exception of water and salt, are organic ingredients. Products labeled "organic" mean that 95 percent of the ingredients are organically produced. Lastly, "made with organic ingredients" on a food means that at least 70 percent of the product is made from organically produced ingredients.

In my 14 years of clinical practice, I have found that the number one predictor of whether or not people choose organic foods is price. The cost of organic items tends to be higher than their conventionally produced counterparts and thus may be a deterrent for many individuals and families. In my mind, a good rule of thumb is to choose your organic foods wisely. There is a list of foods referred to as "The Dirty Dozen" that tend to have the highest level of pesticides. If you are considering venturing into the world of organic foods, this would be a great place to start.

Furthermore, if there are items that your household uses frequently, such as milk, then perhaps that is a worthwhile food to buy organic as you are potentially exposing yourself

The Clean 15
Onions
Sweet corn
Pineapple
Avocado
Asparagus
Sweet peas
Mango
Eggplant
Cantaloupe (domestic)
Kiwi
Cabbage
Watermelon
Sweet potatoes
Grapefruit
Mushrooms

or your loved ones to toxins multiple times a day. It is also worth noting that when we purchase foods from other countries, we are eating foods from places where legislation regarding pesticide levels is often lax or nonexistent. When local varieties are available, they are likely a safer choice. On the positive side of things, the Environmental Working Group, which publishes The Dirty Dozen, also offers its recommendation for the "Clean 15." These lists change slightly each year, as pesticide use is somewhat dependent on climate, therefore differing each season.

Genetically Modified Foods

If you are unfamiliar with genetically modified foods or genetically modified organisms (GMO), you may think you stepped 100 years into the future in this section. The truth is that about 90 percent of the foods we ingest every day have some genetically modified organism in them. Genetic modification of crops has been used for decades to create different and improved versions of many species. The main objective of using this technology is to make crops more sustainable, improve taste, reduce cost, and improve farming efficiency. Controversy swirls around this subject due to the lack of labeling of such practices, as well as the potential for allergic reactions and other long-term health risks not researched yet. At this point, the FDA has not mandated labeling of GMO foods but such legislation is likely not far away.

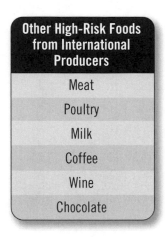

Other High-Risk Foods from International Producers
Meat
Poultry
Milk
Coffee
Wine
Chocolate

Health Claims

The very last thing that you may notice on the packaging of your favorite foods are health claims. The FDA allows for three main types of health claims, as follows:

1. Nutrient content claims ("good source of calcium" or "fat-free")
2. Health claims ("Calcium and vitamin D as part of a balanced diet, along with physical activity, may reduce the risk of osteoporosis.")
3. Structure function claims ("Antioxidants maintain cell integrity.")

These claims are regulated by the FDA and are based on wide bodies of research that have shown that such nutrients do indeed impact our health in the ways described. Use these types of health claims as reinforcement for your already great choices.

It's Time to Shop

You have done your due diligence and are ready to begin your first informed shopping trip. Remember that you are not alone in the aisles of the grocery store. Your grocer is willing and able to assist you on your mission. Do not be afraid to ask a manager at your market for a particular brand or item that you cannot locate. Most stores will be happy to find and order different items if they know there is an interest.

Give yourself plenty of time to do your shopping. When I guide my clients through the market, I always have them show me what they would usually buy and then we examine the food label. If the choice no longer seems ideal, we look above and below that item to see if a healthier version exists. Thanks to the progressive nature of our food industry, there often are healthier alternatives. When you are shopping on your own, you should feel empowered to do the same type of hands-on research. Do not settle for satisfactory nutrition! It is your privilege and right to find food that nourishes and nurtures your body.

Avoid shopping on an empty stomach. Without fail, our choices are skewed in a negative direction when we shop hungry. I think you will find it easier to make great choices if you follow this golden rule. My favorite time to shop is either first thing in the morning after I've exercised and eaten breakfast or late at night after dinner. The aisles of the grocery store tend to be quiet at these times, affording me the time I need to read and explore.

Lastly, I know those of you who shop for a family likely

try to avoid bringing your kids along with you to the grocery store as it tends to belabor the process. I would recommend that you occasionally bring the kids along so that you can begin to impart the important nutrition lessons you have learned. There are a multitude of teachable moments in the grocery store that most parents do not take advantage of. Give them math assignments based on the nutrition facts label of a particular food, or have younger children pick out all of the colors of the rainbow in the produce section. Teaching young children that good nutrition is fun, delicious, and easy is invaluable.

Now it is time to enter the automatic door of the grocery store and begin your quest toward good health. Take your time, remember your key principles, and have fun. Oh yeah, and do not forget your reusable grocery bags. According to the EPA, one million plastic shopping bags are discarded every minute worldwide, costing companies 4 billion dollars and irreversibly damaging our environment.

Part Two

An Aisle-by-Aisle Guide

Your method for approaching your regular grocery shopping is simple. Use your new knowledge to read and understand food labels, and choose products that you know will satisfy both your taste buds and your quest for good health. As I walk you through the aisles of your market, note that certain products will gain my highest commendation, while others fall short for various reasons. I will highlight products in each category of food, whether it be potato chips or salad dressing, that I feel taste great and are beneficial for you.

The foods that I believe should win a spot in your weekly grocery cart will be will be awarded an **Everyday Eats** designation, as I feel they can be enjoyed daily as part of a healthy lifestyle. Those foods that I feel can be enjoyed in moderation will receive an **Occasional Eats** designation.

In an attempt to make eating healthy a positive experience, I will not list foods that I feel you should avoid. In fact, I truly believe there is no such thing as a bad food, but rather poor habits that get most people into trouble. I will, however, highlight potential pitfalls in each aisle to keep you on track. Make every attempt to focus on fitting in the healthy foods rather than eliminating the lousy ones. When you approach the journey toward healthy eating from this positive place, it feels and works better. You now possess the knowledge to determine which foods simply do not fit into your new way of eating.

Perfect Produce

The produce section is clearly the promised land of the grocery store, the place where every choice is a good one and you can let your guard down a bit. It is here that your goal is to choose as much produce as will fit in your refrigerator and your budget.

Key Food Facts

Vitamins and Minerals: Fruits and vegetables are our greatest nutritional bank of both vitamins and minerals. Often times, you can identify which vitamins are present in produce simply by the color. By choosing a variety of fruits and vegetables each day, you are sure to provide your body with the vitamins and minerals it needs. In the United States, the recommended daily intake of fruits and vegetables is 5 servings per day. This number is significantly fewer than the number recommended by other governmental agencies. For example, Canada's food guide recommends adult males get 10 servings of fruits and vegetables per day. The moral of the story is to try to consume as many servings of fruits and vegetables as possible.

Fruit and Vegetable Colors and Nutritional Content	
Red	Lycopene, ellagic acid (mostly found in berries, pomegranates, and walnuts), and quercetin. Act as antioxidants to reduce cancer risk, lower LDL cholesterol, and lower blood pressure.
Orange and Yellow	Beta-carotene, flavonoids, lycopene, potassium, and vitamin C. Reduce cancer risk, lower cholesterol and blood pressure, and promote healthy joints and healthy immune system.
Green	Fiber, thiamine, riboflavin, niacin, vitamin E, lutein, zeaxanthin, calcium, magnesium, folate, vitamin C, calcium, and beta-carotene. Antioxidants boost immunity, lower cholesterol, and support healthy vision.
Blue and Purple	Resveratrol, vitamin C, fiber, flavonoids, ellagic acid, and quercetin. Boost immune function, aids digestion, lowers cholesterol, and limits cancer cell activity.
White	Lignans (phytoestrogens), beta-glucans, EGCG (potent antioxidant common in green tea), SDG (lignin common in flaxseed), and folic acid. Powerful immune modulators, decreasing cancer risk and balancing hormone levels.

Sugar: You may have heard that carrots are very high in sugar, or that sweet potatoes are not good for you because they are high in sugar. The truth is that, yes, fruits and vegetables are natural sources of sugar, but I have never met anybody who gained a lot of weight from eating too many carrots. Have you?

The sugar content of produce is often offset slightly by the natural fiber content of the fruit or vegetable. I would never avoid a type of produce because of concerns for sugar content.

Fiber: You should rely heavily on fruits and vegetables to provide dietary fiber at meals and snacks. See the Produce Fiber chart to learn how your favorites stack up in terms of their fiber content.

Produce Fiber Chart Food	Serving Size	Fiber (g)
Apple	1 medium	4.4
Asparagus	½ cup cooked	1.7
Avocado	1 medium	13.5
Banana	1 medium	3.1
Beets	½ cup	2.5
Blackberries/boysenberries/raspberries	1 cup	7.6
Blueberries/strawberries	1 cup	3.6
Broccoli	1 cup	8.0
Brussels sprouts	¾ cup	3.0
Cantaloupe	1 half	2.0
Carrots	½ cup	3.4
Celery	½ cup	4.0
Corn	1 medium ear	5.0
Cucumber	10 slices with skin	.7
Eggplant	2 thick slices	4.0
Grapefruit	1 medium	2.5
Grapes	1 cup	1.4

Produce Fiber Chart Food	Serving Size	Fiber (g)
Greens	1 cup	8.0
Guava	1 cup	8.9
Kiwi	1 medium	2.1
Mango	1 medium	3.7
Mushrooms	5 small	1.4
Nectarine/peach/plum	1 medium	2.4
Orange	1 medium	3.1
Papaya	1 cup	2.5
Pear	1 medium	5.5
Peas	½ cup	9.1
Peppers	½ cup	2.0
Pineapple	1 cup	2.3
Pomegranate	1 medium	11.3
Potato	1 medium	4–5.0
Squash	½ cup	3.0
Tomato	1 medium	1.5
Watermelon	2 cups	1.1
Yams	1 medium	6.8

Choosing Ripe Produce: Fruits fall within one of two categories when it comes to ripening. Climacteric produce will continue to ripen after it has been picked. This list includes avocado, peaches, bananas, apples, melons, plums, and tropical fruits. Non-climacteric fruits are those that reach their peak ripeness while still on the tree or vine. This list includes berries, citrus fruit, cherries, dates, and grapes. Do not buy a package of strawberries that are barely red and hope they will reach their full potential once they get home. What you see is what you get when it comes to non-climacteric produce. It is okay to purchase an unripe avocado and let it rest on your kitchen counter until it is soft and ready for use.

Think of the following four characteristics to determine the freshness of produce:

- **Color** is often a great indicator of the level of ripeness. Look for consistent coloring all over the fruit.
- **Weight** Ripe fruits tend to be heavier than less ripe varieties. This is because as the produce ripens it gets juicier, thereby making it heavier.
- **Texture** should be consistent all over the piece of fruit.
- **Flavor and Aroma** A full aroma should be present but not overwhelming. Smell fruit at the end opposite the stem to determine if it is worthy of purchasing. When produce is refrigerated it may be more difficult to use aroma as a good indicator.

Organic: Many consumers are torn between choosing typically more expensive organic produce and sticking with the less expensive conventionally farmed offerings. Whatever is going to help you sleep better at night is really the best answer on this topic. If you want to stretch your dollar and only choose some organic produce, check out a list referred to as "The Dirty Dozen" (see page 52). This is a compilation of the 12 fruits and vegetables that are most likely to have high levels of pesticide residue. Because of climate changes each year, this list varies from season to season. Visit www.ewg.org/foodnews to review the Environmental Working Group's up-to-date list of pesticide levels. As a general rule of thumb, consider organic produce when you intend on eating the skin of that product (apple, peach, plum), and stick with less expensive products when it comes to things you are going to peel (oranges, bananas, watermelon).

In Season: Locally grown fresh produce tastes good. There is just something significant about knowing that your apple was grown up the road, loaded on a truck, and sold at your grocery store. Less romantic is the premise of choosing grapes, for example, that were farmed in Mexico, distributed to large food distribution companies throughout the United States, and then driven by truck or train to your grocery store days, weeks, or months later.

In our culture, we expect to be able to buy peaches in December and apples in June. Nutritionally speaking, there is really nothing wrong with that plan. Sure, the apple you eat 6 months after it was picked may be slightly less nutrient-dense, but it does not mean that is not good for you. If you hope to buy only fresh-in-season produce, look for tags at the market that indicate where the produce was grown. Oftentimes the employees in the produce section are terrific resources to help you choose locally grown fare. You can also check out www.fruitsandveggiesmorematters.org for a full list of in-season produce.

Storage: Different recommendations exist for the storage of different types of produce. Root vegetables, including onions, pumpkin, squash, turnips, and parsnips, should be stored at room temperature. Other vegetables can typically last for about one week in the refrigerator. It is not a good idea to wash produce prior to storage. Moist produce can be wrapped in paper towel to help absorb some of the moisture and prevent sogginess. Apples, bananas, nectarines, and melons should not be stored near other produce. As they ripen, they omit gases that can cause other fruits and vegetables to ripen too quickly.

Pitfalls

Any choice you make in the produce section is a good one. In my experience, it seems the one pitfall people experience is simply lack of variety. Most shoppers buy the same types of produce each week because they are comfortable with them and know how to cook and enjoy them at home. I encourage all of my clients to become a bit more adventurous when shopping for produce. Using web sites such as www.eatingwell.com allows you to search for a healthy recipe using just about anything you would find at your market.

Everyday Eats: Produce is the best thing to include each and every day. Remember, we are aiming for 5 servings of fruits and vegetables each day as a minimum. That usually works out to either a fruit or a vegetable each time you eat. This will not only help to ensure you are receiving proper vitamins and minerals, but it will help you meet your fiber needs as well.

Insider Tips

- Roast Vegetables—by far my favorite way to enjoy just about any vegetable. There are two main ways I like to roast vegetables.

  1. Quick Vegetable Roast: Place a single layer of your vegetable of choice on a baking sheet. Asparagus, sliced zucchini, mushrooms, and onions work well in this format. Use a small amount of olive oil and a dash of kosher salt or other seasoning and lightly cover the veggies (a Misto—oil sprayer available at Bed Bath & Beyond—is a great way to spread olive oil on veggies for roasting). Bake veggies at 400° for about 20 minutes or until they reach your desired level of doneness.

  2. Slow Vegetable Roast: Use a large roasting pan or disposable aluminum pan. Fill up the pan (about 3 inches high) with your favorite concoctions. I love Brussels sprouts, parsnips, turnips, onion, whole garlic cloves, broccoli, squash, carrots, and diced white and sweet potatoes. Again, use a small amount of olive oil and kosher salt to toss the veggies. Bake in a 350° oven for 2–3 hours, stirring occasionally. These vegetables come out so sweet and perfect you will not believe that they are good for you. Use leftovers for the next two days as toppings on salads and sandwiches.

- Kabobs are a wonderful way to enjoy vegetables as well. Either on their own or mixed with chicken, beef, shrimp, or salmon, these fast-cooking skewers make for a complete dinner that is fun to eat.

- Combine your fruits and veggies into delicious salads. Try slicing fresh fruit into your next spinach salad. It is beautiful to look at and savory to eat. Strawberries, mangos, grapes, apples, and pears are my favorite additions to any salad.
- Use veggies in place of chips for dips such as salsa or hummus. Using dips is a nice way to get everyone, including picky kids, to begin a love affair with fresh produce.
- Bring your produce with you! You are not likely to eat that much fresh fruit and vegetables if you do not have it around. Pack baggies full of cut-up veggies to take to work and school each day.
- Make produce easily accessible. If you have kids, they will always defer to a packaged snack in the pantry if the produce is not cut up and easily reached. The same is true for most adults. Take a few minutes to make sure the produce you purchased is ready for consumption.

Bottom Line

Study after study indicates that diets high in fresh fruits and vegetables are good for us. Those diets lower our blood pressure, cholesterol, and cancer risks. Fruits and vegetables also give us energy, keep our GI systems regular, and take the place of other less healthy snacks. Plan to include fresh produce as often as possible as part of a balanced diet.

Bountiful Breads

For much of my career, the word bread has almost been given profanity status. Anyone who has attempted a weight-loss plan within the last decade has likely sworn off bread and other bread-like products in an attempt to lose those bothersome pounds. Well, the truth of the matter is that the right types of bread can be a wonderful addition to your food choices.

In fact, researchers from Spain's La Paz University studied 122 women for 16 weeks. The women were divided into two groups. Each group practiced positive lifestyle modifications and received nutrition education. The one difference between the two groups was that one group was allowed to eat bread and the other was not. The results showed that weight loss between both groups was similar and that the group that was allowed to eat bread stuck to the assigned diet more effectively than the no-bread group. The obvious conclusion—

when we like our diet we stick to it! Incorporating great whole grain bread and bread products is a terrific way to make your diet satisfying.

Key Food Facts

Fiber: When shopping for breads, fiber is the most important thing to consider. Each slice of bread should offer at least 2 grams of fiber. If you are choosing products for small children, 1 gram of fiber per slice would also be acceptable.

Calories: A typical slice of bread is around 80 calories per serving. Many bakeries offer light bread options that have a lean 40 calories per slice. These are awesome alternatives if you are attempting to follow a calorie-controlled diet. There are also a number of products available, including sandwich thins and bagel thins, that sport a low 100 calories per serving, which is terrific.

Sodium: Did you know that breads are a major contributor of sodium to our diets? While there is not much you can do about the sodium content of commercially prepared bread products, it is important to note the higher sodium content of many bread products if you are attempting to eat a very low-sodium diet. If you are looking for lower-sodium breads, try brands such as Ener-G, Food for Life, Natural Ovens, and Nature's Way. Most commercial breads contain about 130 mg of sodium per slice. That may not sound like a lot, but the amounts add up over the course of the day if bread is a staple at your meals.

Serving Size: If you are going to make a sandwich, you need 2 slices of bread, right? For most regular breads, that equates to about 160 calories. If you are attempting to follow a somewhat calorie-controlled diet, that does not leave much room for other food at lunch. As an option, you could choose a light bread for your sandwich, which saves half the calories. Recently, I have become a big fan of skinnier bread-type products that offer fewer calories and a satisfying consistency for around 100 calories. Take note of the serving size when purchasing breads to determine if you are getting enough bang for your buck.

Pitfalls

- Whole wheat does not always mean whole grain, and whole grain does not always mean that there is fiber in there. We cannot rely on the title of the bread to indicate if the product is a great one. There are multiple whole wheat breads that have zero grams of dietary fiber and, similarly, there are white breads that actually do have fiber. Be sure to always read the Nutrition Facts to determine the nutrient density.
- "Gluten free" does not necessarily mean healthy. While gluten-free breads are terrific for those who are gluten sensitive, they do not offer tremendous health benefits for the rest of the population. In fact, they are often higher in calories and fat than gluten-containing alternatives.

Everyday Eats: Whole grain breads, bagels, wraps, and pitas are a great way to add fiber into anyone's diet. In my family we have become reliant on some outstanding bread products that taste great and are good for you.

Product	Calories/ Serving	Fiber (g/serving)
Flatout Light Wraps	90	9
Aunt Millie's Hearth Whole Grain Hamburger Bun	110	7
Thomas' Bagel Thins	110	5
Arnold Sandwich Thins	100	5
Arnold Pocket Thins	100	5
Aunt Millie's Hearth Whole Grain Hot Dog Bun	80	5
Boboli Whole Wheat Thin Pizza Crust	120	4
Food for Life Ezekiel 4:9 Bread	80	3
Aunt Millie's Light Potato & Fiber Bread	35	2.5
Ian's Panko Whole Wheat Breadcrumbs	70	2

Occasional Eats: Traditional breads, including French bread, sourdough, rye, and challah, fall into this category. While I recognize that these types of bread are likely not going to be eliminated completely from our diets, I would encourage you to make them more of an occasional eat. If you are going to choose bread that does not have any fiber in it, be sure to enjoy it as part of a fiber-full meal. Also, be sure to avoid overdoing it on the bread basket before you begin your main meal. Choosing these types of bread are likely to make you hungrier at the meal, which leads to overeating.

Insider Tips

Use some new products to make easy and filling meals and snacks. Try using a light Flatout for a breakfast sandwich. Simply take two hard-boiled eggs, dump the yolks, break the high-protein egg whites into a few pieces and lay them on the wrap. Sprinkle with reduced-fat shredded mozzarella cheese and microwave or toast until the cheese melts. Add a slice of tomato or a dollop of ketchup if you like, roll up the wrap, and you have a high protein, high-fiber egg white breakfast sandwich to go. Total prep time is about 90 seconds!

For a satiating snack, use one Thomas' Bagel Thin to create a healthy pizza bagel. Spread a small amount of marinara sauce and reduced-fat shredded mozzarella cheese on top and toast or microwave until ready. This is the perfect after-school snack as it is appealing and filling at only about 150 calories.

Arnold Pocket Thins are the perfect canvas for just about anything. Add a few slices of turkey and spread some hummus inside for a delightful and light sandwich. Fill with 2% cottage cheese, sprinkle with cinnamon, and heat for about 20 seconds for a sandwich with the taste of a crepe and a fraction of the calories.

Use healthy potato and fiber bread to make egg-white French toast that anyone would enjoy. Purchase a carton of egg whites for dipping the bread and use a non-stick cooking spray to limit saturated fat. Top with sliced strawberries and enjoy!

Makeover Moments: Make over your next meal by swapping new bread finds for old habits. Even your favorite sandwich will thank you!

White bread turkey sandwich	= 250 calories	0 g fiber
Arnold Pocket Thin turkey sandwich	= 190 calories	6 g fiber
Your savings	60 calories	**Your gain** 6 g of fiber

A bagel with cream cheese is a popular, yet relatively unhealthy choice. See what happens when we swap a regular bagel with regular cream cheese for a bagel thin with light cream cheese.

Regular bagel with cream cheese	= 400 calories	21 g fat	2 g fiber
Bagel thin with cream cheese	= 170 calories	4 g fat	5 g fiber
Your savings	230 calories	17 g fat	**Your gain** 3 g of fiber

Bottom Line

Americans like bread! So why not incorporate several high-fiber products to slim the profile of your daily diet? You will notice that fiber containing grains offer substantially more satisfaction than the refined varieties and that you feel better eating them.

Deli Delicious

There are tremendous treasures to be found behind the glass of the deli counter if you know what you are looking for. Deli meats can include everything from whole cuts of meat to chopped varieties. They can provide a low-calorie source of protein in many instances. The deli counter is also the home to sliced cheeses and dozens of prepared salads, soups, and meal starters. Uncovering the healthiest offerings among the various options can make waiting in the deli line well worth your time.

Key Food Facts

Sodium: The sodium content of most deli meats is extremely high. Even regular turkey can have sodium levels around 230 mg per ounce, which translates to a sandwich that has over 1,000 mg of sodium or half of your day's allowance. If sodium is a concern, look for low-sodium varieties, such as Hillshire Farm's lower-sodium turkey and ham, Applegate Farms no-salt turkey, Dietz & Watson no-salt turkey, and Meal Mart sliced meats.

Nitrates: Most deli meats use some form of nitrate as a preservative. Nitrates act to prohibit bacterial growth, including dangerous botulinim. Nitrate consumption has been linked to the formation of nitrosamine, a known carcinogen. For this reason, consuming excessive amounts of nitrates in your diet is not recommended. It is worth noting that food production techniques have advanced over the years to include ascorbic acid in foods which require nitrates, which helps to prevent the dangerous conversion of nitrates to nitrosamines. If you would rather play it safe, nitrate-free deli meat can be found at your deli counter and should be chosen if such foods are a regular part of your diet. Look for brands such as Dietz & Watson, Hormel Naturals, and Applegate Farms for nitrate-free deli options.

Saturated Fat: Saturated fat is the type of fat that is found in meat and high-fat dairy products. Choosing full-fat varieties of deli meat and cheese can add an unhealthful amount of saturated fat to our daily diets. Always look for reduced-fat options at the deli counter. Soft cheeses tend to have lower amounts of total fat than hard cheese. Once you have made your selection, be sure to ask for things to be thinly sliced. This will keep serving sizes small and thus keep saturated fat intake to a minimum.

Prepared salads tend to be laden with saturated fat as well. The healthiest ingredients can be a diet mishap when they are combined with high-fat mayonnaise.

Organic: Choosing deli meats with an organic designation indicates that the meat was raised in an environment free of antibiotics, hormones, and pesticides. Applegate Farms offers organic, all-natural options for the discriminating shopper.

Shelf Life: Once you pick up your items at the deli counter, it is important to note that the shelf-life of these items is not particularly long. Any prepared dish should only be kept in the refrigerator for up to two days, and sliced deli meat is safe in the fridge for up to five days. Be sure to keep these items at temperatures below 40 degrees and to avoid allowing them to sit outside of the refrigerator for more than two hours.

Pitfalls

One could really lose their way when shopping at the deli counter in a sea of over 300 different items. Keep an eye out for high-sodium, higher-fat options that offer little in the way of nutritional benefits.

- Limit sectioned or formed meats. While these products tend to be budget friendly, they are not particularly healthy. These items are formed from various cuts of meat and meat by-products stuck together with other additives and fillers. Formed meats tend to be higher in fat and sodium than whole cuts of deli meat.
- Bacon is a staple in many families. Seek out the leanest cuts, and watch frequency of consumption. Choosing lean turkey bacon or lean Canadian bacon in place of regular bacon can save calories and fat grams. Jennie-O and Applegate Farms offer healthier

nitrate-free alternatives for occasional consumption.

- Ask your dedicated deli counter staff which choices are lower in sodium and nitrates in order to make the best possible choice. Try to substitute poultry-based options for traditional beef- and pork-based products in order to save on calories and total fat.

- Do your research ahead of time. When you are waiting in a long line at the deli counter is not the time to start comparing labels of various brands to determine the best choice. Check out your favorite brand's web site prior to shopping so that you can compare food labels. Also, web sites like nutritiondata.com or calorieking.com will allow you to search for a particular brand name and learn about its nutritional composition.

- Prepared soups run the gamut from extremely healthy to extremely not! Look for broth-based soups that have plenty of vegetables and beans in them. I love minestrone or lentil soup as a lunch or even a snack. Cream-based soups, unless labeled low in fat, are typically full of saturated fat from full-fat milk or heavy cream. These items should be avoided on a regular basis.

- When purchasing deli salads, be aware of creamy dressings and fattening preparations. Often times a dish may sound healthy, like "layered eggplant," yet the preparation of that item likely would include frying of the eggplant. The same thing goes for tuna vegetable salad or spinach dip. While some of the ingredients may be healthful, their combination with full-fat mayonnaise makes them undesirable for your waistline. Instead, look for deli items that are grilled, and salads that are labeled low- or no-fat.

- Keep your eyes open for new and flavorful combinations of ingredients with which you are not familiar. Trying something such as a quinoa (keen-wa) salad from the deli counter may motivate you to purchase quinoa on your own and become creative.
- Read your labels. The words used to describe a particular item can be deceiving. Be sure to browse the ingredient list and look for fillers or other additives. For example, "chicken sausage" may have a lot of other things in it besides chicken!
- Frequency and Quantity. If you are purchasing organic, nitrate-free, lower-sodium deli meat, then you are in great shape. Use these foods as great low-calorie healthy options to add to lunches and snacks as a source of protein. If, however, you are purchasing whichever bologna is on sale that week, consider how often and how much you include these foods. Diets high in processed meats have been linked to increased incidence of gastric cancer.

Everyday Eats: I applaud the food manufacturers who have come to the rescue of all the busy people in this country by producing high-quality, high-nutrition products that are safe for us to enjoy regularly. Go ahead, give them a standing ovation. These foods receive an everyday eats exemplary award for their convenience and healthfulness.

Product	Serving Size	Calories	Total Fat (g)	Sodium (mg)	Nitrate Free (Y/N)
Dietz & Watson Lower-Sodium Turkey	2 oz	50	0.5	330	Y
Dietz & Watson Uncured Classic Dinner Ham	2 oz	60	2.5	440	Y
Applegate Farms Organic Roasted Chicken	2 oz	60	1.5	360	Y
Alpine Lace Reduced-Fat Cheese	1.2 oz	110	7	75	Y
Grilled chicken	3.7 oz	120	1.5	670	Y
Grilled vegetables	1 cup	35	0.7	13	Y
Quinoa salad	1 cup	100	5	104	Y
Lentil soup	7 oz	130	3.5	580	Y

Occasional Eats: Conventional deli meats, and by that I mean those with nitrates and no low-sodium designation, receive an occasional eats designation. I like the fact that even these products can offer a low-calorie source of protein that is easy to use and easy to find. I certainly understand that we all have budget and time constraints that impact how and what we eat. Choosing reputable brands and monitoring frequency and portion size makes lean deli meats a nice option once or twice a week. Similarly, hot dogs are a large part of the culture in this country. Rather than recommending that my clients never eat a hot dog, I recommend choosing lower-fat varieties every once in a while.

Product	Serving Size	Calories	Total Fat (g)	Sodium (mg)	Nitrate Free (Y/N)
Hebrew National Reduced Fat Beef Franks	1 hot dog	120	10	360	N
Boar's Head Sliced Turkey	2 oz	60	1	350	N
Jennie-O Extra-Lean Turkey Bacon	2 slices	40	1	240	Y
Low-fat cheese	1 oz	110	7	75	Y
Low-fat spinach dip	2 oz	130	9	580	Y
Grilled vegetables	1 cup	35	0.7	13	Y
Chicken noodle soup	13 oz	120	1.5	1380	Y
3-Bean salad	3.5 oz	90	4.5	480	Y

Insider Tips

It bears repeating that it is essential to combine a good source of protein with a fiber-full carbohydrate each time we eat. For many people, using healthy deli meat is a terrific way to add that lean protein to any meal or snack. I like adding shaved, lean deli turkey meat to the top of a salad, creating a whole grain wrap with turkey slices, hummus, and a wedge of avocado, or simply wrapping a slice of turkey around a slice of fruit.

- Roll up a few slices of healthy turkey and use in between fruit on a kabob.
- Shaved turkey makes a great filling for a lettuce wrap. Simply take a few leaves of iceberg lettuce to use as a breadless wrap and fill with your favorite concoction. I love mixing shaved turkey with diced mango, diced

avocado, diced tomato, and a drop of balsamic vinegar. You can even premake these wraps and serve them as an appetizer at your next get-together.

- Reduced-fat hot dogs are the perfect start for "hot dog, hamburger, and fries kabobs" that adults and kids will enjoy. Cut the hot dog into 1″ pieces and place them on a skewer alternating between grape tomatoes, frozen potato wedges, cubes of pineapple, and turkey meatballs. Simply place on the grill or on a broiling pan and dinner is ready in 10 minutes.

- Enjoy soups for snacks. Often we choose a snack that we can eat while we run around and do a million things. The problem with this is that we never slow down to actually realize what it is we are eating. Choosing soup as a snack requires you to sit at the table and pay attention to your food. When we pay attention to what we are tasting, we make more suitable choices.

Makeover Moments: If you are used to buying full-fat deli meats and cheeses, you will be amazed at the amount of calories, fat, and sodium you can save by making over your deli choices.

Food	Calories	Fat (g)	Sodium (mg)
3 slices salami with 1 slice American cheese and mayo on white bread	497	30.6	1508
3 slices low-sodium turkey with 1 slice of low-fat Swiss cheese and mustard on whole wheat bread	370	10	800
Your savings	127	20.6	708

Change how you grill at your next barbeque by changing the type of hot dogs you serve to your family and guests.

Food	Calories	Fat (g)	Sodium (mg)
Bratwurst on white bun	380	23	880
Reduced-fat hot dog on whole wheat bun	200	10	500
Your savings	180	13	380

Bottom Line

It is ideal to choose foods that are as whole and natural as possible. That said, unless you have an unlimited amount of time and resources, chances are you are going to have to rely on the convenience and ease of items from the deli from time to time. By making educated choices in this category, you can feel good about including healthful deli meats, soups, salads, and low-fat cheese in your daily menu. Keep your discriminating eye on labels for total fat, sodium content, and ingredient lists. The fewer additives and preservatives, the better.

Going Fishing!

If your expedition for good health does not stop at the fish counter, you are likely on the wrong path. Seafood provides a tremendous source of protein that is naturally low in saturated fat and high in healthful omega-3 fatty acids. It is advised that most people try to eat two to three 4-ounce servings of fish per week. Consumers are often intimidated by fish because they do not know how to prepare it, or they are turned off by the odor or consistency of raw fish. With a few great recipes, adding fish into your diet can be easy, affordable, and delicious.

Key Food Facts

Mercury: Mercury is a mineral often found in detectable concentrations in seafood. The mercury content of fish varies greatly from one type of fish to the next and is dependent on the fattiness of the fish, as well as the way it was raised (farm-raised or wild). It is a good idea to choose fish that are considered to be lower in mercury on a regular basis. This is an especially important recommendation if you are pregnant, nursing, or feeding young children. The effects of mercury contamination are increased in the growing tissue of children's brains. The Center for Disease Control (CDC) and the Environmental Protection Agency (EPA) have teamed up to provide the following recommendations with regard to safe seafood consumption:

- Do not eat shark, swordfish, king mackerel, or tilefish because they contain high levels of mercury.
- Eat up to 12 ounces (two average meals) a week of a variety of fish and shellfish that are lower in mercury. Five of the most commonly eaten fish that are low in mercury are shrimp, canned light tuna, salmon, pollock, and catfish. Another commonly eaten fish, albacore ("white") tuna has more mercury than canned light tuna. When choosing your two meals of fish and shellfish, you may eat up to 6 ounces (one average meal) of albacore tuna per week.
- Check local advisories about the safety of fish caught by family and friends in your local lakes, rivers, and coastal areas. If no information is available, eat up to 6 ounces (one average meal) per week of fish you catch from local waters, but then don't consume any other fish during that week.

Omega-3s: Omega-3s are types of fat that have almost medicinal qualities. Acting as street cleaners, omega-3

Type of Fish	Total Omega-3 /3.5 oz. Serving (g)
Mackerel	2.6
Trout, lake	2.0
Herring	1.7
Tuna, bluefin	1.6
Salmon	1.5
Sardines, canned	1.5
Sturgeon, Atlantic	1.5
Tuna, albacore	1.5
Whitefish, lake	1.5
Anchovies	1.4
Bluefish	1.2
Bass, striped	0.8
Trout, brook	0.6
Trout, rainbow	0.6
Halibut, Pacific	0.5
Pollock	0.5
Shark	0.5
Sturgeon	0.4
Bass, fresh water	0.3
Catfish	0.3
Perch, ocean	0.3
Flounder	0.2
Haddock	0.2
Snapper, red	0.2
Swordfish	0.2
Sole	0.1

fats sweep through our arteries and veins, helping to keep our cholesterol low and plaque formation to a minimum. Furthermore, omega-3s are the preferred building blocks for brain development. When a woman is pregnant, the preferred type of fat that can be transferred to the fetus is omega-3. Many people who do not include fish in their diet regularly seek out omega-3s in the form of a supplement. Studies support the consumption of omega-3s fatty acids from fish instead of a supplement at least two to three times per week to reap the benefits of a diet high in omega-3s. The FDA recommends that adults receive around 3 grams of omega-3s each day. They further advise that no more than 2 of those grams come from supplements. Research has shown that the absorption and efficacy of omega-3s from fish is superior to obtaining the omega-3 from a fish oil supplement.

Cholesterol: Certain seafood, including shrimp, tends to be higher in cholesterol than one would think. A high-cholesterol diet is just one factor that contributes to high cholesterol in your blood. If you have been diagnosed with high cholesterol, then it is advised that you keep total daily cholesterol intake to less than 200 mg per day. One 3.5 ounce serving of shrimp has 200 mg of cholesterol. However, the other cardiovascular benefits of choosing a diet high in fish may outweigh any concern about having shrimp or other seafood as part of a healthy diet.

Farm-Raised: Farm-raised fish are those that are typically bred in contained areas on the shores of large bodies of water. There are a number of environmental and health concerns related to farm-raised fish. The often overcrowded conditions at many fish farms are the potential breeding ground for a number of issues, including the increased risk of infection, need for antibiotic use, and elevated levels of toxins including polychlorinated biphenyls (PCBs) in the water due to large amounts of fishmeal and excrement. Furthermore, fish farms may have a negative impact on the greater environment when some fish are able to escape and interrupt spawning in the natural environment. I advise my clients to choose wild fish whenever possible, or to limit farm-raised fish to one serving per week. If you enjoy fish but have a difficult time finding wild varieties, try canned wild salmon.

Wild: Wild fish is often the preferred way to go when purchasing seafood, but you cannot let your guard down completely when you see the word "wild" on your favorite fish. Many fish are caught using techniques that are damaging to the environment and the species of fish themselves. Overfishing has caused several types of fish, including Chilean sea bass, to become endangered. Moreover, unsafe fishing practices lead to a tremendous amount of waste on a global scale. To make the smartest fish purchases, look for a seal of approval from organizations including the Marine Stewardship Council, Fishwise, or Seafood Safe. These organizations allow you to make educated choices in terms of benefits-versus-risks associated with various types of fish.

Shelf Life: I prefer to purchase fresh fish on the day I intend to use it, but fish can be kept in the refrigerator for 48 hours before you prepare it. If you are planning on cooking fresh fish, it is a good idea to purchase fish on a day when you know there was a fresh delivery to the store. For example, most stores do not receive fresh food deliveries on Sunday, so I would try to not purchase fresh fish on a Sunday. Luckily, most stores offer terrific frozen fresh fish options that allow you to enjoy the health benefits of fresh fish every day of the week for a fraction of the cost! Try Costco fresh salmon filets from the freezer or Trader Joe's frozen fish varieties. At a regular grocery store, check your freezer for single-serving frozen fish pieces that can be defrosted and prepared quickly and healthfully. Lean fish can be kept in the freezer for up to six months, and fatty fish can be frozen for two to three months.

Pitfalls

It is pretty hard to go wrong nutritionally at the fish counter. How you prepare the fish, on the other hand, can make or break your seafood meal. Frying or sautéing fish adds a lot of unnecessary fat to your dish. Topping fish with high-calorie tartar sauce can also take away from an otherwise healthy meal. Broil, bake, poach, or grill your favorite fish with your favorite seasonings.

- Salmon filet (two pounds for family of 5) Lemon juice, lime juice, sprinkle kosher salt, cover with parsley flakes and reduced-fat parmesan cheese. Bake at 375–425° until cooked through and then broil to brown cheese on top.

Everyday Eats: For adult consumers who are not pregnant or nursing, choosing fish regularly is an excellent choice. If you are purchasing food for children, or you yourself are pregnant or nursing, your seafood consumption should be planned out so as not to exceed the recommended intake of 12 ounces per

Type of Fish	Calories 3 oz.	Mercury (ppm)	Omega-3 Content (g)
Wild Alaskan salmon	175	0.014	1.88
Chunk light tuna	99	0.118	1.6
Cod	89	0.095	0.150
Mackerel	114	0.05	2.390

week. The FDA action level for mercury is 1.0 ppm. You can see in the chart that these safe fish choices offer the benefits of omega-3s without the harmful levels of mercury.

Occasional Eats: It is advised that certain fish only be consumed occasionally because of the risk for mercury contamination. These fish still offer many nutritional benefits, including the fact that they are a lean source of protein and healthful omega-3 fats. Choose these fish every once in a while to add variety and flavor to your regular diet.

Type of Fish	Calories 3 oz.	Mercury (ppm)
Yellow fin tuna	92	0.08
Swordfish	103	1.226
White or Ahi tuna	90	0.86

Insider Tips

Often the simplest preparations for fish are the most enjoyable. If you are short on time, simply top your piece of fish with your favorite seasonings and broil for 10–12 minutes.

Many kids rank fish pretty low on their favorites list. Try these ideas to make eating fish more fun.

- My kids' favorite way to enjoy salmon is when it is marinated in a combination of soy sauce and brown sugar. This tangy concoction seems to give the fish just the right flavor for diners of all ages.
- Make a fish sandwich. Add a little low-fat tartar sauce or ranch to a fish sandwich on a whole grain bun and watch your kids warm up to the idea of having fish for dinner.

- Try pretzel or Goldfish Crackers–encrusted tilapia or cod. This baked crunchy dish is sure to please even the pickiest of eaters.

Ingredients

4 (⅓ lb.) filets tilapia or other white fish

1½ cups crushed Goldfish Crackers

1½ cups shredded reduced-fat cheddar cheese

½ cup whole wheat flour

½ tsp. salt

½ tsp. pepper

½ tsp. paprika

½ tsp. onion powder

½ tsp. garlic powder

4 egg whites, beaten

Non-stick cooking spray

Rinse and pat dry the fish filets. Combine dry incredients in a shallow dish. Coat fish in egg whites and then dredge in dry ingredients. Place on a baking sheet sprayed with non-stick spray.

Bake at 350° for 15–20 minutes and enjoy!

Substitute fish for chicken or meat in a familiar recipe. Fish tacos or a Greek salad topped with salmon are examples of easy ways to incorporate fish into a regular meal. Enjoy adding other seafood including shrimp, clams, flounder, crabs, and scallops for low-mercury options.

To keep fish affordable, look for sales at your local market or buy fish in bulk from a warehouse store and freeze it in individual portions for easy use at a later date. Canned tuna and salmon are also relatively budget-friendly options. Tilapia, whitefish, and cod tend to be less expensive fresh options and they are easy to cook and prepare.

Try making a healthy tuna noodle casserole. By using low-fat Italian dressing, whole grain pasta noodles, and some added vegetables such as peas and mushrooms, you can create an entire meal in minutes.

Tuna Noodle Casserole Recipe

Ingredients

1 box whole-grain pasta noodles

2–3 oz. can of albacore tuna

1 can baby peas

1 can sliced mushrooms

1 can crushed pineapple in its own juice

⅓ cup low-fat Italian dressing

2 Tbsp. low-fat mayonnaise

1 bag reduced-fat shredded mozzarella cheese

Directions

Cook pasta until ready to eat.

Mix tuna and mayonnaise to make tuna salad.

Combine drained pasta, tuna salad, peas, mushrooms, and pineapple in 9 x 11″ glass dish.

Toss with Italian dressing. Top mixture with shredded reduced-fat mozzarella cheese.

Bake at 350° for 20 minutes. Broil for last 5 minutes or until cheese is browned on top.

Food	Total Calories	Saturated Fat (g)	Omega-3 Fat (g)
6 oz. steak with mashed potatoes and creamy spinach	516	12	0
6 oz. salmon with 3 oz. baked sweet potato and steamed asparagus	420	4.3	4
Your savings	96	7.7	**Gain** 4 grams omega-3

Makeover Moments: Just changing two meals a week from meat or poultry to fish can help you achieve an improved cardiovascular risk profile. By substituting high saturated fat entrees like steak with high omega-3 dishes like salmon, you will make your body happy.

Bottom Line

Do your homework and dive into the world of fresh fish as a terrific alternative to other animal-based proteins. If you are in a group at high risk for mercury contamination, be sure to monitor your intake to keep levels within safe parameters.

Making Meat Matter

If following a vegetarian lifestyle is not for you, it is important to learn how to make meat and poultry a healthy part of your diet. Meat is an excellent source of protein and important micronutrients, including iron, vitamin B12, zinc, phosphorus, magnesium, and selenium. Poultry is similarly nutritionally robust in that it provides a quality source of protein, selenium, and B vitamins including niacin.

Key Food Facts

Often times we purchase meat and poultry from a counter at our grocery store. These items are not always wrapped in packaging that displays their nutritional information. For this reason, you must know what you need and want before you place your order. Think of these key food facts when determining which meat and poultry to purchase:

- **Extra-Lean** applies to several cuts of meat including

round roast and top sirloin steak. These cuts have less than 5 grams of total fat, 2 grams of saturated fat, and 95 milligrams of cholesterol.

- **Lean** According to the USDA, there are 29 cuts of meat that qualify as lean. The USDA defines "lean" as fewer than 10 grams of total fat, 4.5 grams or

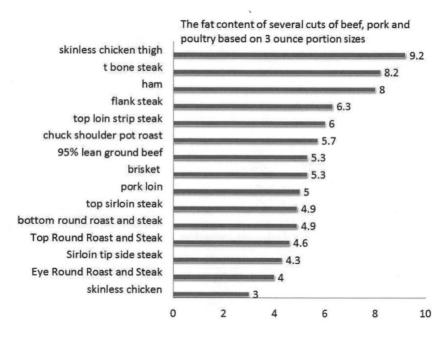

The fat content of several cuts of beef, pork and poultry based on 3 ounce portion sizes

Cut	Fat
skinless chicken thigh	9.2
t bone steak	8.2
ham	8
flank steak	6.3
top loin strip steak	6
chuck shoulder pot roast	5.7
95% lean ground beef	5.3
brisket	5.3
pork loin	5
top sirloin steak	4.9
bottom round roast and steak	4.9
Top Round Roast and Steak	4.6
Sirloin tip side steak	4.3
Eye Round Roast and Steak	4
skinless chicken	3

fewer of saturated fat, and less than 95 milligrams of cholesterol per 3-ounce serving. These numbers are similar to that of a boneless, skinless chicken breast. Choosing from the list of lean meats is an excellent place to start when purchasing beef.

- **Grain-Fed** The majority of meat that is available in commercial grocery stores is grain-fed. This means that for the majority of the animals' lives they are eating grass in the pasture, but for the last 3 to 6 months the animals are brought into the feedlot and given high-energy grain to speed their growth. This process tends to produce a marbling and flavor enhancement to which most Americans have become accustomed.

- **Grass-finished or grass-fed** beef is being found more often in grocery stores around the country. This type of beef comes from animals that are allowed to feed on the grass in open pastures for their entire life. It is thought that this way of raising animals for beef is better for the consumer, the animal, and the environment. Grass-fed beef tends to be more costly and has a slightly different flavor and texture than grain-fed beef.

- **Natural** is defined by the USDA as all animals raised for human consumption without additives and minimally processed. All fresh meat is natural.

- **Organic** is defined by the USDA as animals born and raised on certified organic pastures, free of antibiotics and hormones, fed diets of solely organic grains and grasses, and with unrestricted outdoor access.

- **Free-Range** is another USDA definition that means poultry have been allowed access to the outdoors. Of interest is the fact that this designation does not imply anything about the amount of time spent outdoors, or the conditions or quality of that outdoor space.

- **No Antibiotics Added** is a label claim also regulated by the USDA. It means that the animal was raised without the use of antibiotics.
- **Certified Humane** is a voluntary distinction offered by outside agencies. Certified Humane meat producers adhere to elevated standards related to every process of animal care from birth to slaughter.

Pitfalls

Common pitfalls at the butcher counter are easy to avoid with new food labels and nutrition knowledge. As of January 2012, the FDA is mandating that most meat and poultry products wear a nutrition label. Packages of ground meat and poultry as well as 40 of the most popular cuts of meat will have nutrition fact panels that display all of the nutrition information that you will need to make an educated choice, including calories, total fat, saturated fat, and cholesterol per serving. These labels also require food manufacturers to not only state the percent lean but also the percent fat of the package. For example, if the meat is 80 percent lean, it also has to say that it is 20 percent fat. This new level of transparency will be helpful in preventing consumers from making poor choices.

Poultry vs. Beef vs. Pork A common pitfall in this aisle is the assumption that a poultry or pork-based product is necessarily more healthful than a beef product. For example, a 4-ounce serving of ground turkey (85 percent lean) provides 266 calories and 15 grams of fat, 4 of which are saturated.

A similar serving of lean ground beef (95 percent lean) provides only 193 calories, 7.4 grams of fat, and 3.4 grams of saturated fat. I would guess that nine out of ten consumers would automatically assume that the ground turkey is the better choice, when it fact it is not. Similarly, many cuts of pork are just as lean as poultry. In fact, 6 cuts of pork meet the USDA guidelines for "lean." Be sure to read past the name of the product to determine what is your best choice.

Avoiding the meat counter all together. Many consumers avoid the meat counter altogether in efforts to improve their cardiovascular health and or lower their cholesterol. Many times, the first piece of advice physicians give their patients when treating high cholesterol is to cut back or avoid meat. The truth of the matter is that obtaining and maintaining an ideal body weight is the best way to impact both cholesterol levels and overall health. By choosing healthy, lean meat and poultry, many consumers are able to build a diet that is both low in calories and very satisfying. This combination is likely to help consumers achieve their goals of reaching a healthy weight. If you are not a vegetarian, I would encourage you to include lean meat and poultry in your regular diet.

Everyday Eats: When I am building diets for my clients, I love to include white meat poultry, and lean ground poultry and beef, as they are relatively low in calories and provide a very satisfying source of protein that tends to inhibit excessive snacking throughout the day. Enjoy adding these favorites into your daily menu.

Food	Calories 3 oz. serving	Total Fat (g)	Saturated Fat (g)
White meat chicken without skin	142	3.0	0.9
White meat turkey without skin	91	1.1	0.4
95% lean ground turkey	122	6.1	1.9
95% lean ground beef	145	5.6	2.5
Sirloin	160	5.6	2.1
Eye round roast	148	5.3	1.9

Occasional Eats: Other cuts of beef and poultry are less desirable on a day-to-day basis because of their higher fat content. These foods should only be eaten occasionally in efforts to keep cholesterol levels in check and your arteries and veins clear.

Food	Calories 3 oz. serving	Total Fat (g)	Saturated Fat (g)
Filet mignon	152	5.6	2.1
Chicken wing	247	16.6	4.6
Ground beef (85% lean)	183	12.8	5.0
Ground turkey (85% lean)	200	11.2	2.9

Insider Tips

- The USDA offers guidelines on the purchasing and safety of various meats. Visit http://www.ams.usda.gov /AMSv1.0/getfile?dDocName=STELDEV3002633 for a complete meat buying guide (or simply go to usda.gov and search "meat buying guide").

- When you purchase and prepare meat and poultry, be sure to trim visible fat and remove skin. These components add a large amount of total and saturated fat to any meal.

- Shelf life: Ground meat and fresh poultry can be kept in the refrigerator for 1–2 days and in the freezer for up to 4 months. Fresh cuts of meat can remain safely in the refrigerator for 3–5 days and in the freezer for up to one year. For best results, wrap pieces of meat individually. Cooked poultry can be enjoyed from the refrigerator for 3–4 days or frozen for about 4 months. Be sure to store cooked food in shallow pans to allow for safe cooling.

- Watch cooking methods. Baking, broiling, boiling, or grilling are typically your best bets. One of my easiest dinners is made with boneless, skinless chicken breasts, a bottle of low-fat French dressing, a bag of baby carrots, and a package of mushrooms. Simply mix and bake in a 350° oven for about 1.5 hours. It will not disappoint!

- Perhaps my favorite tip for those new to healthy shopping and cooking is to transition to lean ground turkey for everything. Okay, maybe not everything, but there are seemingly endless uses for ground white meat turkey. Turkey burgers, turkey meatballs, turkey meatloaf, turkey spaghetti sauce, turkey chili, turkey tacos … you get the point! The texture of the lean turkey can be intimidating at first as it is somewhat sticky when you are trying to form burgers or meatballs, but trust me, once it cooks it is quite perfect.

Turkey Meatloaf (serves 4)

Ingredients

1 lb. ground white meat turkey

2 egg whites or 1 whole egg

½ cup seasoned bread crumbs

½ cup ketchup

¾ tsp. salt

½ tsp. black pepper

1 Tbsp. minced onions

3 cloves garlic or 1 Tbsp. minced garlic

Directions

Mix all ingredients in a large bowl. Press into a loaf pan and bake at 350° for about 1 hour.

- If you enjoy certain cuts of meat that do not fall into the lean or extra lean category, have them in small servings occasionally. Controlling portion size is a wonderful way to enjoy all foods in moderation.

Makeover Moments: Your favorite dinner can take on a completely different look by substituting leaner ground turkey or beef in your next recipe. See the magic for yourself.

Food	Total Calories	Total Fat (g)	Saturated Fat (g)	Dietary Fiber (g)
Spaghetti with ground beef (85% lean) and regular enriched pasta (3 oz.)	623	13.5	5.0	0
Spaghetti with lean ground beef (95% lean) and whole grain pasta (3 oz.)	500	6.0	2.5	15
Your savings	123	7.5	2.5	**Your gain** 15

Bottom Line

Educated consumers can make lean meat and poultry a healthy part of their daily diet. Make choices that reflect both your viewpoints on farming and agriculture and your desire to watch calories and fat. Most importantly, make enough for leftovers! Already cooked meat and poultry is an easy-high protein topping for a salad the next day at lunch.

Shall We Can-Can?

The first few years I was on my own in the kitchen I relied heavily on the ease and convenience of canned foods. I mean, canned foods are sort of hard to beat. All you need is a can opener and dinner is on the table. It is estimated that up to 17 percent of the U.S. diet is composed of canned foods, so I guess I was not alone in my reliance of this form of fast food.

In recent years, however, a spotlight has been placed on the canned food industry and bisphenol A (BPA), specifically. BPA is an industrial compound that is used in the lining of food and beverage cans. Independent and government agencies have acknowledged that BPA has been linked to a number of health concerns, including cancer and reproductive issues. The FDA and U.S. Department of Health and Human Services are currently examining new research on the safety of BPA in our food supply. Concerns regarding BPA toxicity are highest in young children and pregnant and nursing moms. If you fall into that category, you may want to take extra caution when choosing canned foods.

Key Food Facts

Sodium: Most canned foods use sodium as a flavor enhancer and preservative. If you are following a low-sodium diet, it is not advisable to choose canned foods. One serving of canned green beans has 400 mg of sodium. That is nearly a quarter of your daily allowance if you are on a low-sodium diet. Thankfully, many food producers have begun to offer low-sodium varieties of your favorite canned goods. It is also effective to rinse canned foods in a strainer prior to use. This will help to remove a great deal of the original sodium content.

Calcium disodium EDTA is commonly used in canned goods as a preservative and to help foods retain color. This additive is considered safe by the FDA, but studies are ongoing as to its potential effects on the gastrointestinal system. If you find you are sensitive to food additives, choosing to avoid canned goods with added calcium disodium EDTA is likely a good decision.

Monosodium glutamate (MSG) is found in certain canned foods. Many people are extremely sensitive to MSG in foods and should read ingredient lists on canned goods in efforts to avoid it as an additive.

Fat: Many canned soups are cream based and have upwards of 10 grams of fat per serving. Look for soups that are broth-based instead. Those tend to be lower-fat options. Oftentimes, a soup may sound healthy like tomato soup, for example, yet the Nutrition Facts panel will reveal an unnecessary amount of added fat.

Pitfalls

As a realistic registered dietitian, I acknowledge that the convenience and budget-friendly nature of canned goods is hard to pass up. So what is a consumer to do when they are faced with concerns about the safety of their food supply? In my mind, moderation is a key concept. If you are using canned food here or there, then levels of potential unhealthy ingredients are unlikely to add up to anything of consequence. If, however, you rely heavily on canned food, it is probably a good idea to take a second look at your grocery cart and see how you may be able to substitute fresh or frozen produce for canned goods.

Everyday Eats: Perhaps the only food from the canned food section that I see the benefit of including every day is beans. Beans are a super food of sorts in that they contain valuable dietary fiber as well as provide a good source of vegan protein. Cooking and preparing raw beans is a time-consuming process that does not always allow for consumers to enjoy them whenever they would like. That makes choosing canned beans a true nutritional treasure. Rinse them in a strainer to remove excess sodium and potential preservative residue and add them to soups and salads regularly.

Occasional Eats: Canned vegetables and healthy canned soups could be enjoyed in moderation as part of a healthy diet.

- Look for low- or no-added salt varieties of vegetables. There is often a savings of nearly 250 mg of sodium per serving.
- When shopping for soups, look for broth-based soups that have plenty of vegetables and beans. Seek out organic canned soups to ensure an added level of healthfulness. My favorite is Trader Joe's Organic Lentil Soup.
- Although these are not traditionally in a can, pickles are typically found in this section. While pickles do not have any caloric impact on our diet, they are very high in sodium, often rounding out at near 1,000 mg per pickle. Limit these in your regular diet.

Insider Tips

- Use your canned food allowance wisely. If you are attempting to limit canned foods, choose those that are hard to find fresh or frozen. Enjoy things like artichoke hearts, hearts of palm, beans, and high-quality soups.
- Substitute fresh or frozen vegetables for common canned vegetables, including green beans, carrots, corn, and mushrooms.
- Choose food stored in glass jars in place of canned foods to avoid potential BPA toxicity.
- Purchase beverages in more environmentally friendly packaging whenever possible.

Makeover Moments: Making over your canned food choices is less about changing total caloric intake and more about changing how you shop and think about food. Having said that, look how great these easy swaps look in your pantry.

Food	Calories	Sodium (mg)
Green beans	20	400
Low-sodium green beans	20	200
Your savings	0	200

Food	Calories	Fat (g)	Fiber (g)
Chunky clam chowder	230	13	3
Lentil soup	160	2	5
Your savings	70	11	**Gain** 2

Bottom Line

Think moderation and ease of preparation when prioritizing which canned goods to add to your grocery cart. If you are able to limit your reliance on these types foods, you will be that much closer to a diet comprised of mostly whole, unadulterated foods, which is a good goal.

Classy Condiments

Would there even be a point to eating if you could not dip, spread, or marinate? In my mind, choosing the right condiment can make all the difference in the world in terms of both flavor and nutritional profile. A good friend of mine cannot eat anything that has sauce on it, so she has nothing to worry about in this aisle. For the rest of the ranch dressing–loving, barbeque sauce–dipping readers, you are not going to want to miss the next few pages.

Key Food Facts

Fat: Many spreads, dressings, and marinades are high in fat. Oils are made completely out of fat. While label reading, be sure to take note of the type of fat in a certain product, as this is how you will determine if it is a good choice or a must-skip. Peanut butter, for example, is high in fat (16 grams/2 tablespoon serving), but if you notice on the label, only 3 grams of that 16 is saturated fat, meaning the other 13 grams are heart-healthy mono- and polyunsaturated fats.

Look for low-fat varieties of salad dressings and marinades when possible. On average, a swap from regular to low-fat dressing saves 10 grams of fat per 2 tablespoon serving. I prefer to choose the low-fat variety instead of the fat-free variety most of the time simply because I think it tastes better and tends to have less artificial additives and preservatives.

Sugar is somewhat of a hidden ingredient in certain salad dressings and sauces because you do not expect it to be there. Most store-bought sauces and salad dressings have added sugar in them to enhance flavor. Read labels and raise eyebrows if sugar content is greater than 10 grams per serving. To take it one step further, check similar products on the same shelf to see if you can find one that does not have a lot of added sugar.

Condiments, including jelly and jams, can also be found in lower-sugar varieties. One tablespoon of regular jam has about 50 calories and 13 grams of sugar. A tablespoon of low-sugar jelly has half the calories at 25 and only 5 grams of sugar. This is a significant savings in terms of calories and sugar grams. To put these numbers in perspective, remember that one teaspoon of sugar is 4 grams. Now would you rather have three teaspoons of sugar on your toast or only one? Seems like a pretty simple question to me. Smucker's Low-Sugar Preserves have no artificial sweetener in them either, making them a safe choice for the whole family.

Calories: It would be a shame to take a healthy meal like a salad or a chicken breast and ruin it by adding a whole lot of calories. This is a very common mistake that many individuals make. Take a grilled chicken salad, for example. The salad itself is likely around 300 calories, but when you add 4 tablespoons of ranch dressing to it, the salad becomes a 700-calorie choice. Look for dressings, sauces, and spreads that have between 50–120 calories per 2 tablespoon serving. This will help to keep your calories in check.

Sodium: Many marinades and salad dressings are high in sodium. Two tablespoons of my favorite barbecue sauce have around 300 mg of sodium. Two tablespoons of ketchup have 320 mg of sodium as well. That is a lot if you are watching your salt intake. Look for lower-sodium options, including Lum Taylor's Low-Sodium BBQ Sauce or Walden Farms lower-sodium dressings and marinades. Heinz also has a fantastic no-salt ketchup that has only 10 mg of sodium in the same two tablespoon serving.

Pitfalls

The condiment aisle is not a place to fall down on the job. The proper selections of sauces or spreads will require label reading in the beginning. Be sure to compare similar products to find the best fit for your needs. Some of you will stick to the low-sodium options, while others are primarily focused on choosing lower-sugar varieties. Be aware that when food manufacturers take away an ingredient, such as salt in a low-sodium product, they often add in another ingredient, in its place to make up for the change in flavor. Often, lower-fat options will be slightly higher in sugar. With some trial and error, I am confident you will find the condiment that fits your needs best.

Everyday Eats: The list of condiments that can be enjoyed every day is quite long. Healthy condiments are often the best way to add a great deal of flavor without adding a lot of calories. Check out these options while perusing the condiment aisle on your next grocery store visit.

- **Peanut Butter:** I think the best bet is to go for a natural product when possible. Jif's relatively new Omega-3 Peanut Butter is a unique product and excellent way to get essential fatty acids, DHA and ARA, into the diet of non-fish-eaters. If calories are your main focus, seek a peanut butter substitute that offers about half of the calories of regular peanut butter.

Food	Calories 2 Tbsp.	Total Fat	Sugar (g)	Sodium (mg)
Jif Reduced Fat Peanut Butter	190	12	4	220
Better 'n Peanut Butter	100	2	2	190
Jif Omega-3 Peanut Butter	190	16 (8 g mono)	3	150

- **Jelly and Jam:** When possible, look for products that are made from fruit and are lower in sugar. Using smaller serving sizes is also a great way to keep calories and sugar intake to a minimum in this category.

Food	Calories/Tbsp.	Sugar (g)
Smucker's Low Sugar Jelly	25	5
Smucker's Simply Fruit	40	8

- **Ketchup and Mustard:** America's two favorite condiments, ketchup and mustard, deserve to have a place in your grocery cart. Mustard is naturally very low in calories. Each serving has fewer than 5 total calories, making it a guilt-free addition to anything. Ketchup often gets a bad rap for being high in sugar. Have you ever met anyone that gained a lot of weight from eating a lot of ketchup? I have not! So unless you are filling your plate up with ketchup daily, I do not suspect ketchup will be a problem in your diet profile. If you do seek to cut out added sugars altogether (regular ketchup has about 4 grams per tablespoon), there are no-added-sugar varieties on every grocery store shelf.

Food	Calories/Tbsp.	Sugar (g)
Ketchup	15	3.4
Mustard (yellow)	3	0
Dijon mustard	15	0
No-added-sugar ketchup	5	1

- **Hummus:** This refrigerated product made from chick peas, olive oil, and tahini (sesame seed oil) is a must for me. It is relatively low in calories and packs a lot of flavor. My favorite way to enjoy hummus is with veggie sticks. Look for hummus in individual packs, as well as larger containers for week-long dipping enjoyment!

- **Barbecue Sauce:** Choosing that perfect flavor for your next dinner is critical. Keep these helpful tips in mind when you are reading labels on this finger-licking category. Limit artificial ingredients including high-fructose corn syrup, keep sodium levels below 300 mg per serving, and carbohydrates less than 10 grams.

Food	Calories 2 Tbsp.	Total Fat (g)	Sugar (g)	Sodium (mg)
Whole Foods 365 Organic BBQ Sauce	100	8	6	260
Annie's Naturals Organic BBQ Sauce	45	1	5	220
Consorzio Organic BBQ Sauce	45	0	9	280
Dinosaur Bar-B-Que Sensuous Slathering Sauce	25	0	5	240
Kraft Light Barbecue Sauce	20	0	3	340

- **Salad Dressings and Marinades:** Did you know that your body is more able to absorb many of the nutrients from your favorite salad if there is some fat in your salad dressing? With a small amount of fat present, your body has to produce enzymes to break it down. These enzymes help your body to absorb the fat-soluble vitamins (vitamins A, D, E, and K) that are present in various vegetables. Look for light or low-fat varieties that are bursting with flavor. If you prefer salad dressing from the bottle, I find the best flavors for low-fat dressings are French, Italian, or vinaigrette. Read ingredient lists and limit brands with added high-fructose corn syrup, artificial colorings, and preservatives. Often when the number of fat grams in a serving of salad dressing goes down, the number of sugar grams goes up. Be aware of higher sugar options that do not contribute to the healthfulness of your diet.

Food	Calories 2 Tbsp.	Fat (g)	Sugar (g)	Sodium (mg)
Kraft Light Raspberry Vinaigrette	50	3.5	5	240
Ken's Light Options Balsamic Vinaigrette	60	4.5	4	210
Ken's Light Options Ranch	80	7	2	310
Newman's Own Lite Honey Mustard Dressing	70	0	5	280
Mrs. Dash Salt-Free Spicy Teriyaki	50	1	6	0
Newman's Own Lite Low-Fat Sesame Ginger Dressing	35	1.5	4	330
Newman's Own Teriyaki Marinade (1 Tbsp)	25	0	4	330
Newman's Own Herb & Roasted Garlic Marinade (1 Tbsp)	20	1	2	370

• **Mayonnaise:** There are basically three options when it comes to mayonnaise. First is to go for the full-fat variety, which I do not recommend. I mean, why choose a product that has twice the fat when there is an equally tasty product sitting right next to it that has half the fat? The second choice is to select the reduced-fat or low-fat types that tend to maintain a familiar mayonnaise taste with about half the fat. The last option is pick a fat-free mayonnaise. On their own, the fat-free spreads have a somewhat artificial taste and may be a turn off to those new to eating healthy. If you want to try a fat-free spread, I recommend doing so when there are lots of other flavors present, including, but certainly not limited to, mustard, spices, hummus, or ketchup. Using a small amount of reduced-fat mayonnaise or Miracle Whip can help you to create beautiful salads made with tuna, egg white, or chicken.

Food	Calories 2 Tbsp.	Fat (g)	Sugar (g)
Miracle Whip Light	25	1.5	2
Light mayonnaise	49	5	0.7
Miracle Whip Fat-Free	15	0	2
Fat-free mayonnaise	13	0.4	1.6
Kraft Mayo with Olive Oil	45	4	1

• **Oils:** Any endorsement I make when it comes to oils should not be misconstrued as a license to deep fry anything! Certain oils are healthy when they are used in small quantities. Choosing oils that are higher in mono-unsaturated fats to use in cooking or for salad dressings is a good idea for both your palate and your heart!

Food	Calories Tbsp.	Fat (g)	Saturated (g)	Mono-unsaturated (mg)
Extra virgin olive oil	119	14	2	9.8
Canola oil	119	14	1	8.3
High oleic sunflower oil	124	14	1	11.7
Hemp seed oil	130	14	1.5	1.3

- **Vinegars:** Typically a very low-calorie way to add the perfect splash of flavor to just about anything. Balsamic vinegar clearly wins the popularity contest when it comes to these fermented liquids. Balsamic is perfect on a salad or as part of a marinade. Other vinegars include apple cider vinegar, white vinegar, rice vinegar, red wine vinegar, and white wine vinegar. Vinegars can last on your shelf for up to two years, but, once opened, should be used or disposed of within three months. It is fun to play around with different vinegars as they each embody a different flavor and level of tanginess.

Food	Calories Tbsp.	Sugar (g)	Sodium (mgs)
Balsamic vinegar	14	2	4
Rice vinegar	0	0	0
Red wine vinegar	3	0	1
Cider vinegar	0	0	0

Occasional Eats: I want you to enjoy healthy condiments every day. They are going to enhance your dining experience whether you are eating at home or your desk. The right sauce or spread can really bring your meal to life. If you feel that making the switch to lighter varieties is too much of a challenge for you or your family, consider making condiment use more of an occasional thing instead of an every-meal thing. For example, if you love ranch dressing and typically use it at lunch and dinner on most days, consider making ranch dressing just an occasional food, like once a week. After all, eating healthy is all about moderation. Similarly, if you love ranch dressing, try cutting your portion size in half by mixing one tablespoon of ranch dressing with two tablespoons of salsa. This zippy mix has a fraction of the calories and fat grams.

Insider Tips

- Make your own salad dressings. Simply choose a healthy oil, add in your favorite vinegar and a squirt of your favorite citrus fruit such as orange, lemon, or lime. This fresh and light combination is the perfect complement to any salad.
- Purchase a Misto to cut down on the amount of oil you need to dress a salad. You can find a Misto at your local kitchen supply, online, or at a household-type store. It allows you to spray a thin layer of your favorite oil on salads or vegetables before grilling.
- Check for the type of dispensing top that is provided

with your dressing. An open spout lends itself to more dressing coming out with each use, while a shaker top helps to limit dressing amounts. If you love a certain dressing but not the bottle it comes in, consider transferring it to another container or using a small dish. With the dish, you can cut your calories in half by dipping your fork into the dressing instead of pouring it over the salad.

- Combine your favorite condiments to produce a healthier hybrid. Reduced-fat mayo is lower in fat than regular mayo, but we can make it even better. Mix half reduced-fat mayo with dijon mustard and your next roll up sandwich will thank you.
- Buy a cruet! For those of you who do not know what a cruet is, it is simply a glass bottle with a pouring spout on the top. Good Seasons sells one in most grocery stores with a packet of their Italian dressing seasoning mix (which is very good by the way). I use my cruet to make homemade dressings all the time. There are even markers on the glass bottle so you know how much oil, vinegar, and water to add. To make the dressing lighter, you can add in a bit more water and a little less oil than the markings indicate. I make a combination of balsamic vinegar, canola oil, and two packets of Truvia or Splenda artificial sweetener. Shake it up and you will have the best dressing you have ever tasted.
- Change how you think about dressing your sandwiches.

If you always have mayo on your bread, consider switching to zero-calorie mustard or low-fat mayo instead. You may be surprised how much you enjoy a plain sandwich.

Makeover Moments: A makeover with condiments is easy to illustrate. Once you see the facts, you will never go back!

Meal	Calories	Fat (g)	Sugar (g)
Caesar Salad with 2 Tbsp regular dressing	270	21	8
Caesar Salad with 2 Tbsp reduced-fat dressing	145	1	3
Your savings	125	20	5

Next time you mix up your favorite salad, whether it be tuna, chicken, or egg, remember the magic of lite mayo.

Meal	Calories	Fat (g)	Sugar (g)
1 scoop tuna salad with regular mayonnaise	240	21	2
1 scoop tuna salad with reduced-fat mayo	209	10	2
Your savings	31	11	0

Bottom Line

The bottom line on condiments is use them! If we do not enjoy the taste of our food, we are less likely to stick with eating healthy. Condiments can be a wonderful vehicle for getting children and picky adults to try new foods as well. I'll give in to a couple of tablespoons of light ranch dressing any day of the week if it means my child or client will eat a plate full of vegetables! Make the switch to low-fat varieties so that you can enjoy them every day and look great doing so.

Beautiful Baking

The secret to baking smart is to do so occasionally and, when possible, to modify recipes to make them more healthful. I have always said that I would not want to live in a world that did not include birthday cake. Enjoying sweets and treats in moderation is the key to long-term maintenance of a healthy weight. Research has shown us that people who enjoy their diet are more likely to stick with it. By learning how to make healthful baking choices, you will be able to incorporate the occasional sweet treat without guilt or remorse.

Key Food Facts

Fat: Fat is simply something that comes with many baked goods. If you pick up any mix or container of frosting, it contains fat. Several brands offer lower-fat options, including Betty Crocker Low-Fat Chocolate Brownies. Other mixes can be prepared in a low-fat way by substituting applesauce for oil in equal portions, and two egg whites for each whole egg. These swaps can save up to 20 grams of fat per recipe. When baking from scratch, seek out healthier alternatives to butter and heavy creams. Earth Balance or Smart Balance spreads offer a healthier blend of fats than what you would get in butter or margarine. Try using fat-free half-and-half, soy milk, or almond milk in place of heavy cream. Reduced-fat sour cream should also replace full-fat sour cream in baking.

Sugar: Sugar is also a necessary component of most baking mixes. It is important to remember that sugar is sugar. Whether it is brown or white, refined or raw, the caloric value of sugar is the same from one type to the next. If you are baking from scratch, there are a number of sweeteners you may consider. Many of these can be substituted for sugar in a recipe, and often can help reduce the amount of sugar needed. As more and more consumers are attempting to reduce or eliminate sugar from their diets, a long list of artificial sweeteners has developed. These can sometimes be used in place of part of the sugar in a recipe. It is important to note that many of the artificial sweeteners impart a distinctive flavor to the finished product and are gastrointestinal irritants for many individuals. If baking is an occasional activity in your house, I would recommend using real sugar and enjoying small portions of your favorite baked goods.

Pitfalls
- Be cautious if you find a lower-sugar or sugar-free

Sweetener	Traits	As Substitute for 1 Cup Sugar
Honey	25–50 times sweeter than sugar	Use ¾ cup sugar + 1 Tbsp honey + pinch of baking soda
Maple syrup	60% as sweet as sugar	¾ cup and decrease liquid by 3 Tbsp
Molasses	Dark, strong flavor	1⅓ cup and reduce liquid by 5 Tbsp, reduce no more than half sugar in recipe.
Corn syrup	Used in candy making	Don't substitute
Refined fructose	Sweeter than sugar	⅔ cup
Brown rice malt syrup	Looks like honey	1 cup and reduce liquid by ¼ cup
Fruit juice concentrates	Used in baking	¾ cup and reduce liquid by 3 Tbsp
Stevia Saccharine	200–700 times sweeter than sugar. Sold as Sweet-n-Low.	Only substitute for ½ the sugar in a recipe. 6 packets of Sweet-n-Low for ¼ cup sugar
Aspartame	160–220 times sweeter than sugar. Sold as Equal or NutraSweet.	Not a good substitute for baking
Acesulfame potassium	200 times sweeter than sugar. Sold as Sunett or Sweet One.	Use in combination with sugar. 6 packets for ¼ cup sugar
Sucralose	Made from sugar. Sold as Splenda. 600 times sweeter than sugar.	1 cup. Speeds baking time so watch oven closely

baking mix, as these types of products are often loaded with sugar alcohols (maltitol, sorbitol) that can wreak havoc on your gastrointestinal system. Sugar alcohols have to be identified on the food facts panel, so look for them under Total Carbohydrate. Any product that has more than 2 grams of sugar alcohols will have a high likelihood of causing an upset stomach. Sometimes it is simply okay to enjoy the real thing.

• Portion size can be a pitfall for many when it comes to dessert. It is a good idea to precut or portion out your finished product to help stick to appropriate serving sizes. Do not make a whole tray of brownies if you are the only one that is going to eat them!

Everyday Eats: There are really no products in the baking aisle I would want you to eat every day. These items are designed to be occasional foods at best. If you find that you are craving sweets all of the time, it is a good idea to take a look at your diet quality and begin to explore how you can create more balanced meals that will help to keep your blood sugar stable throughout the day and minimize cravings (see "Method to the Madness").

Occasional Eats: We each have a different definition of occasional. Is occasional once a week, once a month? Ideally, you will begin to cut back on how often you and your family feel the need to indulge in sweets. Many of my clients do well at balancing their intake by choosing one or two times a month that they plan to enjoy various treats. For one person it may be a chocolate chip cookie and for another it may be a scoop of ice cream. The more you plan ahead, the more in control you will feel. When you do decide to enjoy a sweet dessert, explore healthier options.

| HEALTHIER OPTIONS FOR DESSERT | | | | |
Food	Calories	Fat (g)	Sugar (g)	Fiber (mg)
Purely Elizabeth Chocolate Chip Cookie Mix	80/cookie	2.5	7	2
Betty Crocker Low-Fat Fudge Brownie Mix	130/brownie	2	19	<1
Krusteaz Fat-Free Blueberry Muffin Mix	130/muffin	0	15	2
Bob's Red Mill Spice Apple Bran Cookies Mix	120	2	10	3
King Arthur Cranberry Sunflower Granola Bar Mix	140/bar	7	12	2
Baking Ingredients				
Splenda	0	0	0	0
Truvia	0	0	0	0
Cornstarch	30/Tbsp	0	0	0
King Arthur Unbleached White Whole Wheat Flour	100/¼ cup	0.5	0	3

Insider Tips

- Look for easy and delicious ways to substitute fat when you bake. If a recipe calls for butter, substitute half of the amount with an equal amount of applesauce. Just ¼ cup of applesauce in place of ¼ cup of butter will save 400 calories.

- Yogurt may also replace heavy cream or butter in certain recipes. In fact, No Pudge! Brownie Mix calls for the addition of one container of yogurt.
- Buy mini-muffin baking sheets to help keep portion sizes small.
- Choose 100 percent whites or other egg substitute products to replace eggs in many recipes. If a recipe calls for more than two eggs, you may notice an undesirable change in consistency. Two egg whites can replace one whole egg.
- Use fruit, including mashed banana and pureed prunes, to add flavor and texture to some recipes.
- Small servings (as in a teaspoon) of semi-sweet chocolate chips, caramel chips, and peanut butter chips can be used in various recipes or melted and used as a topping for very few calories. I love melting chocolate chips and drizzling over high-fiber popcorn. Simply throw popcorn in a plastic container, drizzle with melted chips, put the lid on, shake, and refrigerate for about 10 minutes so the chocolate hardens.
- Do not be afraid to stray from the instructions on your typical baking mixes. Some rules are meant to be broken and these are perfect ones to break. Try adding one can of diet soda to a regular cake mix for a light and fluffy treat. Choose a caffeine-free diet soda so it can be enjoyed by the whole family.

Makeover Moments: A treat is not really a treat if you feel lousy after you eat it. By making some simple swaps to the way you bake, you can enjoy the occasional treat and feel good about it. Check out these calorie-saving stats.

Food	Calories	Fat (g)	Sugar (g)
Vanilla cake mix made as directed	200	6	19
Vanilla cake mix made with Diet Sprite	160	4	17
Your savings	40	2	2

See how these fast fat fixes pay your diet back!

Food	Calories	Fat (g)	Sugar (g)
1 cup oil	1,927	218	0
1 cup unsweetened applesauce	102	0	22
Your savings	1,825	218	**Your gain** 22

Food	Calories	Fat (g)	Sugar (g)
2 whole eggs	144	9.6	0.4
4 egg whites	32	0	0.4
Your savings	112	9.6	0

A chocolatey choice that is sure to please even your skinniest pants!

Food	Calories	Fat (g)	Sugar (g)
1 Tbsp chocolate chips	70	4	8
1 Tbsp cocoa powder	12	0.7	0.1
Your savings	58	3.3	7.9

Bottom Line

Eating healthy does not mean that you do not enjoy the foods that you eat. This is never truer than in the baking aisle. By making a few simple swaps, and watching portion sizes and frequency of treats, delicious desserts can be a fun part of your healthy way of life.

Super Spices

Playing with spices and seasonings is an amazing way to add calorie-free goodness to any daily dish. Learning which spices go with what can help you to become an extraordinary cook. You will also find that with the proper seasonings, you need a lot less added fat to make your meals delicious.

Key Food Facts

Sodium sulfite: Used as a food preservative. Some people are sensitive to sulfites, so checking the ingredient list makes it easy to avoid.

Silicon dioxide: Acts as an anti-caking agent to keep spices free flowing in their bottle.

Calcium silicate: Also acts as an anti-caking agent to keep spices free flowing in their bottle.

Shelf Life: I noticed the other day that I had a bottle of cinnamon that was manufactured before I was born. I mean, it had to have been my grandmother's at some time. My point of sharing this story is that spices do have an expiration date. McCormick Spice Company offers some terrific tips on how to check for spice freshness. They say to check the color and aroma of the spice to make sure they are still vibrant and effective. They also recommend storing spices away from heat, moisture, and direct sunlight in tightly capped containers. Did you know members of the red pepper family, including paprika and chili powder, will stay fresher in the fridge? Thanks, McCormick! McCormick also offers a spot on their web site where you can type in the code from your spice bottle to see how old it is. For general guidelines, see the chart.

Spice	Shelf Life
Ground spices	2–3 years
Whole spices	3–4 years
Seasoning blends	1–2 years
Herbs	1–3 years
Extracts	4 years (except pure vanilla, which has no expiration)

Pitfalls

It is hard to go wrong in the spice aisle with one exception. If you are watching your sodium intake closely, be sure to limit or avoid those spices that are high in sodium including garlic salt, seasoned salt, sea salt, and celery salt. Salts provide 490 mg of sodium per ¼ teaspoon making the salt shaker a bad idea. Do not get caught up in designer salts that appear healthier than average table salt. The truth is that almost all salts have the same amount of sodium per weight and that there is little scientific evidence to support choosing one type of salt over another. Look for other spices that offer great flavor without the added sodium.

Everyday Eats: Experiment with spices at each meal. They are calorie free and relatively inexpensive when you think about how long they last. My favorites list includes:

- Garlic powder
- Onion powder
- Vanilla extract
- Basil
- Oregano
- Ground cinnamon
- Black pepper
- Parsley flakes
- Mrs. Dash salt substitute and salt-free seasoning mixes
- Seasoning blends, including Italian or garlic and herb

I am also a big fan of the seasoning mixes that are sold in thin envelopes at every grocery store. They make dinner simple and healthy by providing easy-to-follow recipes right on the back of the envelope. Several of them come in low-sodium varieties and my favorite chili packet comes both mild and spicy for differing taste buds. Check out these seasoning packets on your next trip down the spice aisle:

- Guacamole mix
- Chili mix

- Chicken parmesan seasoning mix
- Fajita mix
- Taco mix

Lastly, you cannot leave the spice aisle without picking up a container of McCormick's Bac'n pieces. These low-calorie bacon-flavored nuggets lend a ton of flavor for only 30 calories a tablespoon. They are totally vegetarian, too, making them fun for all!

Occasional Eats: Adding salt to your diet should be something you think about doing in moderation. Even if you are lucky enough to have normal blood pressure, a diet high in sodium is not good for you. Each quarter teaspoon of salt added to your dish adds 600 mg of sodium. If you are on a low-sodium diet, your daily sodium allowance is only 2,000 mg for the whole day. It is a good idea to keep salt to a minimum both in cooking and at the table.

Insider Tips

- If you plan to use whole spices (instead of ground ones), be sure to use them in long-cooking recipes. It takes a long time for the flavors to be released in comparison to ground spices, which can be added toward the end of cooking.
- Add simple spices, such as garlic powder, onion powder, and paprika, to just about anything. I use them in hamburgers, meatloaf, meatballs, and even roasted vegetables.
- Adding a bit of vanilla extract to fruit salad or

smoothies adds a distinctive and appealing flavor.

- Experiment with growing your own herbs. It is easy to find small growing kits for your kitchen. You will love being able to use fresh herbs in all of your dishes. Fresh mint is so delicious on everything from soups to watermelon feta salad.

Watermelon Feta Salad

- Cut up ¼ watermelon into bite-size pieces
- Add ¼ cut reduced-fat feta cheese
- Sprinkle with fresh mint leaf in ¼ inch pieces

Makeover Moments: Slashing the sodium of your favorite dish is simple.

Seasoning	Sodium (mg)
Sea salt	500
Mrs. Dash Original Blend	0
Your savings	500

Bottom Line

Keep fresh, flavorful spices stocked in your pantry at all times. You can take something as mundane as a pound of hamburger meat and turn it into a flavorful feast. Watch your sodium intake while enjoying new and interesting flavors.

Nice Noodles
& Other Grains

Healthy pasta and other grains can be an enjoyable way to incorporate high-fiber carbohydrates into your diet. While most boxed pastas lack a tremendous amount of nutritional benefit, there are certain hidden jewels that can be the basis for a fantastic meal.

Key Food Facts

Fiber: The foods in this aisle are primarily carbohydrate based. When you pick up a box of pasta or any other grain, such as rice, couscous, orzo, or barley, your eye should travel directly to the carbohydrate portion of the food label. Look for at least 3 grams of dietary fiber per serving in high-quality grains. Just because a particular box says "whole grain" or "whole wheat," it does not mean that there is dietary fiber. Most whole wheat pasta will have about 3 grams of fiber per ounce of dry pasta (100 calories), while regular pasta will have 0 grams of fiber.

Enriched simply means that certain nutrients including iron, folic acid, and other B-vitamins, such as niacin, thiamin, and riboflavin, are added back into a product that had lost such

> ### Brown Rice vs. White Rice
>
> Brown rice is a lower-calorie, higher-fiber option than white rice.
>
> Each cup of brown rice has 216 calories and 4 grams of fiber, compared to 242 calories in a cup of white rice and less than 1 gram of fiber.
>
> Brown rice is also higher in vitamins and minerals, including magnesium.

nutrients during processing. Enriched pasta is white pasta. Whole wheat pasta maintains many more of its original nutrients, thus not requiring enrichment.

Buckwheat is a gluten-free grain that is used to make soba noodles. Soba noodles have about half the carbohydrate and calories as regular noodles and can be used as a great gluten-free alternative to regular pasta.

Couscous is a wheat-based product that looks like tiny pellets. It is often sold in easy-to-prepare formulations. Many couscous dishes are lower in carbohydrates compared to regular pasta. Couscous can be found in whole wheat and enriched varieties. Seek out the whole wheat types when possible.

Brown rice pasta is a gluten-free alternative to traditional pasta. Brown rice pasta has nearly the same amount of calories as regular pasta, with slightly less fiber than whole grain pasta.

Quinoa (keen-wa) is a high-protein grain that can be cooked to be used in both sweet and salty dishes. Quinoa has a very impressionable taste, meaning it takes on the flavors of the other foods with which it is served. Serve in the morning for breakfast with slivered almonds and fruit, or serve with stir fry as a rice substitute.

Quinoa Oatmeal Recipe

Ingredients

1 cup skim milk

1 cup water

1 cup rinsed quinoa

1 cup fresh berries

½ tsp. cinnamon

⅓ cup slivered almonds

1 packet Truvia

Directions

Combine water, milk, and quinoa in saucepan. Bring to a boil, reduce heat to medium and cover for 15 minutes. Stir in berries, Truvia, and cinnamon, and top with slivered almonds.

Spelt is a grain from the wheat family. It is commonly being used to make a healthy pasta that offers protein, fiber, and micronutrients including B vitamins, iron, and magnesium.

Orzo is simply small pieces of pasta. Orzo is typically an enriched product, although I have seen whole wheat orzo occasionally.

Pitfalls

- Portion Size. We tend to eat too much pasta at any given sitting, making it a tough food to enjoy in moderation. One-third cup of cooked pasta equates to an 80-calorie serving. When you fill your plate with spaghetti, you are likely having 2–3 cups of pasta, which is six to nine servings. That is 540–720 calories of just noodles, and we have not even added any sauce yet. When you do decide to cook pasta for a meal, be sure to do so in appropriate portions to keep calories under control.

- Don't be fooled by the colors. Pastas come in various colors, but this does not necessarily mean they are healthier. In fact, most of them are not. Read labels for fiber grams before purchasing.

Everyday Eats: Choosing the right grain can be the perfect way to build healthy meals. Look for options that offer at least 3 grams of fiber per serving and contain 200 or fewer calories per cup. There are new products entering the market every day that offer lower-carb alternatives to traditional pastas. Read labels and ingredient lists to be sure the savings of calories are worth it. Tofu shirataki noodles are an example of a great low-carb substitute for pasta. Find them in the refrigerator section of most grocery stores.

Occasional Eats: It is a great idea to incorporate a variety of grains into your diet throughout the week. Different blends of both soluble and insoluble fiber, along with a variety of vitamins and minerals, make choosing unique grains a winning proposition. If you are attempting to limit carbohydrates, choose from the list of Everday Eats (above) a couple of times per week. By incorporating whole grains occasionally you will be able to achieve and, more importantly, maintain a healthy weight.

Food	Calories (cup)	Fiber (g)	Protein (g)
Barilla Plus Whole Wheat Pasta	210	4	10
Ronzoni Smart Taste Pasta	170	5	6
Brown rice	198	2.6	4
Quinoa	222	5.2	8.1
Soba noodles	113	3	6
Near East Wheat Pilaf	170	8	7
Near East Lentil Pilaf	180	8	11
Tofu shirataki noodles	20	<2	1
Wheatberries	320	12	13
Barley	200	10	7
Wild rice	166	3	6.5
Kraft Whole Grain Macaroni & Cheese	260	5	8
Fiber Gourmet Pasta	130	18	07

Insider Tips

Keep portion sizes of grain-based foods small by mixing them with plenty of vegetables.

- Make a quinoa and spinach salad that is sure to delight. Prepare quinoa as directed, toss ½ cup with two cups fresh baby spinach and ¼ cup diced fresh or dried fruit. Dress with a simple balsamic vinegar and oil dressing. For a different flavor, mix in one tablespoon of hummus as dressing.

- Use whole wheat pasta to make a healthy macaroni and cheese. I love using Ronzoni Smart Taste Pasta and Breakstone's 2% Cottage Cheese for a simple week-night recipe. Cook pasta as directed and drain. Add a 16 oz. container of cottage cheese and your favorite vegetables and mix. The result is a high-protein, high-fiber comfort food feast.
- Make healthy egg white–fried rice with plenty of vegetables. Use brown rice, tons of veggies, tofu or chicken, and scrambled egg whites to make a typically unhealthy dish into a very healthy one. I use the 100 percent whites in a carton to make cooking with egg whites simple.
- Add in small quantities of whole grains to soups during cooking. Even something simple such as chicken soup can get a fiber boost from a handful of barley added in 45 minutes before completion.
- Use leftover cooked grains to top tomorrow's lunchtime salad.

Makeover Moments: You will feel the impact of switching from enriched products to whole grain ones in just about everything you do. You will feel less hungry, less bloated, and less tired. Not only do the easy changes change your bottom line, they change your bottom all together!

Food	Calories (cup)	Fiber (g)	Protein (g)
Kraft Macaroni & Cheese prepared as directed	340	2	12
Kraft Whole Grain Macaroni & Cheese prepared without butter and with skim milk	260	5	12
Your savings	80	Gain 3	0

Make your next plate of spaghetti delicious inside and out by using whole wheat pasta and lean ground turkey meat sauce.

Food	Calories (cup)	Fiber (g)	Protein (g)
Spaghetti with meat sauce	550	3	30
Whole wheat pasta with lean turkey meat sauce	408	8	30
Your savings	142	Gain 5	0

Bottom Line

You do not have to fear the pasta aisle at the market any longer. Shop for whole grains with confidence. You and those you shop for will grow to love their distinctive flavor. If you simply do not enjoy the taste of whole wheat pasta, try Ronzoni Smart Taste Pasta that offers the nutrition of whole grain pasta with the appearance and flavor of enriched pasta. When shopping for and feeding children, it is a great idea to get them used to the consistency and flavor of whole wheat pasta at an early age. It will be a healthy habit they will have for a lifetime.

Stirring the Sauce

Finding the soul mate for your whole grain noodle may be more difficult than you think. All spaghetti sauces are not created equal. With varying levels of added fat, sodium, and sugar, it is necessary to take a closer look at the saucy deliciousness we call spaghetti sauce.

Key Food Facts

Sodium: The sodium content of most commercial pasta sauces is around 450 mg per half cup. That is nearly a quarter of your recommended daily allowance of sodium. If you are a sodium watcher, look for low-sodium varieties, such as Prego Heart Smart Traditional Sauce, which has only 360 mg, and Rinaldi ToBe Healthy Garden Vegetable Sauce, which has 290 mg per half cup. If you want to cut the sodium content even further, try mixing half jarred spaghetti sauce with half no-added salt tomato sauce, which has only 40 mg per half cup.

Sugar: Perhaps the least likely place you would expect to find added sugar would be in a jar of tomato sauce, but check the label and there it is! Most commercial brands of spaghetti sauce contain between 5 and 10 grams of added sugar in each serving. That is the equivalent of one to two teaspoons of sugar in each serving. If you are seeking a lower-sugar alternative try Hunts No-Added-Sugar Tomato Sauce.

Calories: The total calories in most jarred sauces ranges from 70 to 100 calories per serving. When calories count, seek out lower-calorie options such as Prego's new Light Smart Traditional Pasta Sauce with only 45 calories per serving.

Pitfalls

- Be wary of Alfredo and other cream- or cheese-based sauces, as they are likely to have considerably more fat and cholesterol than a tomato-based sauce.
- Do not confuse the terms "natural" or "organic" with healthy. Just because something is made with all natural ingredients, it does not necessarily make it a great choice.

Everyday Eats: I could eat pasta sauce on just about anything. I love using it as a topping for grilled fish, as a dip for cooked veggies, or simply on top of my spaghetti squash. Find a brand of sauce that meets your nutritional and taste bud needs and keep it stocked in your pantry for a relatively healthy flavor burst.

Food	Calories (½ cup)	Sugar (g)	Sodium (mg)	Fiber (g)
Prego Light Smart Traditional	45	7	410	3
Ragu Light Tomato Basil	60	9	330	2
Newman's Own Fire Roasted Tomato & Garlic Pasta Sauce	70	5	500	2
Ragu No Sugar Added Light Tomato Basil	60	6	320	2
Rinaldi ToBe Healthy Garden Vegetable Sauce	70	5	330	2
Bertolli Arrabbiata Sauce	60	4	450	2

Occasional Eats: There are a number of cheesy and savory sauces on the shelves of your market that are surprisingly less indulgent that you would expect. Enjoy adding these every once in a while to a favorite dish, or perhaps use them to encourage more vegetable eating in your pickiest eaters.

Food	Calories (½ cup)	Fat (g)	Sugar (g)	Sodium (mg)
Barilla Three Cheese Formaggi Sauce	70	1.5	6	430
Ragu Light Parmesan Alfredo Sauce	60	4	0	320
Barilla Tomato & Basil Sauce	80	3	8	360

Insider Tips

• Make your own sauce with a few simple ingredients. All you need are fresh tomatoes, onion, garlic, tomato paste, olive oil, bay leaf, salt, and pepper. In about 15 minutes you can have a delicious homemade sauce free of any added sugar or preservatives.

- Look for Amore Tomato Paste in a tube to add the flavor of tomato paste to homemade sauces without the preservatives of a canned product.
- Use both homemade and store-bought healthy sauces as a vehicle for vegetable and protein eating. Nobody will notice if you sneak in extra chopped vegetables, high-fiber beans, or lean ground turkey meat.
- If you have an immersion blender, use it to blend sauces and other healthful ingredients together to create a nutrient-dense sauce no one will suspect is packed with all the good stuff!

Makeover Moments: Making your favorite dish just a little bit healthier never tasted so good. Simple substitutions of healthy pasta sauce for fuller fat, higher-sodium varieties is a must, especially when it tastes just as good.

Food	Calories	Fat (g)	Sugar (g)	Sodium (mg)
2 cups enriched spaghetti marinara sauce	440	6	15	1100
2 cups whole wheat pasta with light marinara sauce	397	2	11	600
Your savings	43	4	4	500

Bottom Line

Picking the perfect pasta sauce can be fun and delicious. Add fresh seasonings to make the healthiest sauce meet your taste bud needs and make flavorful, fiberful pasta, fish, and vegetable dishes a weekly dinner delight.

Crunchy Cravings

It is time to tackle the chip aisle. Before you turn the corner at the market you may need to psych yourself up, take a deep breath, and reassure yourself of your goal. The items in this aisle tend to be the ones we want the most, yet benefit us the least. I must admit that I am immediately skeptical when shopping for such items, as healthy choices are more the exception than the rule. That being said, there are several options that can keep snacking tasty and fun.

Key Food Facts

Fiber: If a snack food does not have any fiber in it, chances are it will leave me or my family feeling hungry. The minimum amount of fiber that I am looking for per serving is 3 grams. In fact, by law, food manufacturers are allowed to state that a food is a "good source of fiber" if it contains those important 3 grams.

Fat: Many common snack foods are high in total fat, and often the type of fat is not the most heart healthy. Ideally, chips and popcorn would have a total of fewer than 3 grams of fat, and most of that fat would come from monounsaturated sources.

Sodium: Chips and popcorn do contribute to our overall sodium intake. They even make the top-10 list of salt-contributors to our diet. If you are salt sensitive, watching for amounts greater than 200 mg is a good rule of thumb.

Serving Size: Portion size is of the utmost importance when it comes to choosing snack foods. Crunchy, salty snacks tend to make us want to eat more. I know you did not need to read this book to know that! Just think of what happens when someone opens up a bag of chips. You take a few, and then a few more, and before you know it, the bag is empty. When determining if snack foods deserve a spot in your daily diet, review the serving size of the item you are pondering first and ask yourself if that serving would be satisfying.

Pitfalls

- In the snack food aisle, deceptive labels and food names can lead a consumer down the wrong path. Cleverly tagged veggie chips and straws imply that they are a good choice for kids or adults who are reluctant to choose the real veggies on their own. The deception is that these items contain 7 grams of fat per serving, and the first three ingredients are potato flour, sunflower oil, and wheat starch (not carrots, spinach, and tomatoes as implied). The lesson learned in this example is that just because the name of a product sounds great, it may not be the case.

- Other pitfalls include choosing snacks labeled whole wheat without checking for actual grams of dietary fiber. Many products will boast a certain number "grams of whole grain." This does not necessarily translate into grams of dietary fiber. Be sure to check the label to make sure the choice is a good one.
- The words "natural" or "organic" are also often used commonly on snack foods to imply that a food provides health benefits. Remember, potatoes and oil are natural products, but that does not mean that taking potatoes and frying them equates to a healthy snack. Do not be fooled by these arbitrary terms that aim to confuse you.

Everyday Eats: The best choice in this aisle is usually popcorn, as popcorn is a naturally good source of fiber. I also like popcorn because the serving size is large and thus very satisfying. For the same number of calories as 13 potato chips, you could enjoy two cups of low-fat popcorn, which would clearly be more filling. Already bagged popcorns that are popped with either no oil or a healthy oil are excellent alternatives for snacks.

Lots of other products are hitting the shelves lately that boast "popped" in their name. Oftentimes popped food items are healthy choices as they are not fried or baked, but rather popped. I like Garden of Eatin' Popped Tortilla Chips partly because of their beautiful food label. Only 110 calories and 3 grams of fiber makes them an Everyday Eats. Note that Popchips have fewer calories than regular potato chips, yet they lack the fiber in regular popcorn. Legume-based chips, such as black-bean or lentil chips, also provide healthier alternatives. Any products that are made from beans or lentils have the potential to be great, as both beans and lentils are naturally high in dietary fiber. Combining these types of chips with low-calorie salsa and some low-fat cheese can make a typically high-calorie snack, like nachos, into a great one.

Food	Calories	Fiber (g)	Fat (g)	Sugar (g)	Sodium (mg)
Garden of Eatin' Popped Tortilla Chips	140	3	7	0	140
Trader Joe's Potato Lentil Curls	130	4.5	4	0	380
Orville Redenbacher 94% Fat Free Popcorn (3 cups)	120	4	2	0	240
Boom Chicka Pop Popcorn (3⅔ cups)	130	3	8	0	90
Way Better Snack Simply Beyond Black Bean Chips	130	3	6	0	60
Eat Smart Naturals Honey Whole Wheat Pretzels	110	3	2	3	100
Orville Redenbacher Smart Pop Kettle Korn	140	6	2.5	0	230

Occasional Eats: Lower-fat options, including baked chips and whole grain pretzels, can be used as part of a well-rounded diet. How you use the foods you choose is also of the utmost importance. Incorporating a serving of baked chips into a high-fiber meal that has plenty of vegetables, fruit, and/or beans can be a terrific way to include the foods you enjoy while maintaining a high-quality diet. It is not an ideal choice for most people to snack on baked chips on their own. While these are certainly a better choice than regular chips, they do not contain the fiber that we need in a snack to make us feel satisfied. Choosing baked chips on their own is likely to leave you reaching for more.

Regular potato chips	= 160 calories	10 grams of fat
Baked potato chips	= 120 calories	2 grams of fat
Your savings	40 calories	8 grams of fat

Insider Tips

Substitute homemade kale chips for the chips in your pantry. It is as simple as cleaning and drying a bunch of kale, sprinkling with olive oil and a small amount of kosher salt, and baking in a 400° oven for between 8 and 12 minutes, or until crunchy but not burnt. These nutrient-dense, flavorful treats can be kept in an airtight container for 2 days at room temperature.

I rely heavily on the oven-roasted strips of seaweed sold in individual packages at my local specialty market as a chip substitute. One package, which includes roughly 30 sheets of delicately cooked seaweed, contains only 60 calories and has 2 grams of fiber.

Use veggies in place of chips for commonly enjoyed appetizers and side dishes. Instead of serving chips and salsa or cheese dip, try offering an array of different colored vegetables for dipping. You will not only save quite a few calories in the swap, but you will also increase your vitamin and mineral intake.

Makeover Moments: Makeover your snack food choice by comparing labels on your frequently purchased foods. An easy makeover utilizes regular versus baked chips. Regular potato chips contain 160 calories per serving, and 90 of those calories come from fat. Switching to baked chips saves you 40 calories per serving and 8 grams of fat, or 72 fat calories. If at first the baked chips taste significantly less appetizing than the ones you are used to, have no fear, our taste buds are actually quite impressionable. Most people's taste buds adapt to a new way of eating within six weeks of following a different style of diet, so persevere and keep an open mind.

Regular nachos do not usually make the list of health foods. However, substituting veggies for chips and using low-fat toppings can make nachos a beautiful thing! Try using carrot and celery sticks in place of chips, offer guacamole, salsa, and low-fat sour cream for dipping, and just like magic, your body will thank you for indulging sensibly.

Regular nachos without meat	=300 calories	18 grams of fat
Veggie nachos without chips	=80 calories	4 grams of fat
Your savings	220 calories	14 grams of fat

Bottom Line

Let's face it, nobody ever found the fountain of youth or the secret to weight loss in the snack food aisle. But we do know that people tend to lose weight and maintain that weight loss when they enjoy their diets. There is no sense in pretending that we are not going to choose any snack foods as part of our regular diet, so why not make educated choices? Choose healthful options in smaller quantities as part of a well-balanced meal or snack, and enjoy the crunch that comes with healthy chips and low-fat popcorn.

The Cookie & Cracker Conundrum

Crackers and cookies can be topics of confusion for many shoppers. It seems impossible to avoid them completely, but you really do not have to if you know which ones to choose. As with all other carbohydrate-based foods, we are seeking out the tiny slivers of crunchy goodness that offer up some dietary fiber in as few calories as possible.

Key Food Facts

Fiber: The great majority of crackers and cookies on the grocery store shelf lack dietary fiber in any significant amounts. Unfortunately, if you take a look in your pantry right now, there are likely a number of boxes of common snack foods, including animal crackers, cheese crackers, soups crackers, wafers, sandwich cookies, wheat crackers, and graham crackers, that have little or no dietary fiber. What is also unfortunate is that these items are contributing to unwanted weight gain, constant feelings of hunger, and cravings for both sweet and salty foods. Try setting new standards for crackers and cookies by buying ones that offer at least 3 grams of fiber per serving. Just this small amount of fiber can make your favorite crunchy treat a healthy one.

Sugar: When shopping for cookies, the sugar barometer should remain right at 10 grams of added sugar. The source of the sugar in each product may vary from cane sugar to fruit juice, or high-fructose corn syrup to honey, but the calories per gram of sugar remain the same at 4 calories/gram, no matter the source. Two average sandwich cookies have about 14 grams of sugar. That is more than 3 teaspoons of sugar in each serving. Seek out cookies with less than 10 grams of sugar, such as Kashi's Oatmeal Raisin Flax Cookie with 7 grams of sugar. It is also a great idea to check the ingredient list to see where sugar falls. Ideally, sugar would not be listed in the first four ingredients.

Calories: Most crackers and cookies offer servings that are between 100 and 200 calories. Ask yourself if the serving size described, whether it is 13 crackers or 2 cookies, is a satisfying amount for you. If you know that it would take 2–3 servings to make you feel satisfied, that item may not be the best choice. The premise of the 100-calorie pack is a good one if one pack would be satisfying to you. If a 100-calorie pack of your favorite snack often leads to another pack, then it is really a 200-calorie pack!

Trans Fats: Once upon a time, most crackers and cookies were made with trans fats. This is not the case anymore.

Most major food manufacturers have changed the type of oil they use in baking to eliminate trans fats in efforts to make their products more heart healthy. It is still a good idea to check the label to be sure that no trans fats are in the item you are considering. Trans fats are a type of fat commonly found in margarine, which can increase our LDL (bad) cholesterol and our risk for heart disease. Trans fats are not essential to your health, so your intake of them should be as close to zero as possible.

Fat: It is a good idea to limit added fat in your diet. Look for snack items with 4 grams of fat or less. Furthermore, seek out those products that are low in saturated fat as well. The lower the amount of saturated fat, the better.

Sodium: The largest contributors of sodium to our diets are bread and crackers. If you are sensitive to the sodium content of foods, seek out crackers that have fewer than 200 mg of sodium per serving. I love Kashi TLC Original 7 Grain Crackers, which have only 160 mg of sodium and the important 3 grams of fiber for which I am always looking.

Pitfalls

- False Advertising: Many, and I mean many, crackers and cookies are packaged in ways that imply that they are healthy. Whether it is a green box, or the words "natural" or "organic," "whole wheat" or "whole grain," the food producer wants you to believe that its product fits within your healthy lifestyle. The truth of the matter is that there are very few products in this aisle that truly get my stamp of approval. Certain "reduced-fat" cookies, for example, are a better choice than their full-fat cousins, but that does not mean that they are good. You must read labels on boxes and bags to make a choice that works for you.

- 100-calorie packs have been the rage in grocery stores for the last several years. These portion-controlled pouches offer some of your favorite brand-name snacks in small servings for your enjoyment. Many of them still remain high in sugar and fat, making theircute little packages less cute. Having a 100-calorie pack as a stand-alone snack is probably not a terrific idea because it is not likely to be satisfying. I do see a place for certain 100-calorie packs as part of a healthy school lunch specifically, Keebler Fudge Dipped Sandies as they contain 3 grams of fiber and only 6 grams of sugar.

Everyday Eats: A few standout products make my list of crackers and cookies that can be enjoyed every day. Applaud these brands for stepping up and providing us a snack we can proudly sink our teeth into!

Food	Calories Serving	Fat (g)	Sugar (g)	Fiber (g)
Wheat Thins Fiber Selects Five Grain	120	4.5	4	6
Special K Cracker Chips	110	2.5	1	3
100-Calorie Keebler Fudge Dipped Sandies	100	4	6	3
Reduced-Fat Whole Grain Triscuits	120	3	0	3
Quaker Multigrain Fiber Crisps	110	1.5	6	3

Occasional Eats: Having somewhat sensible choices on hand for the occasional treat is a good idea as well. This helps to make eating healthy fun and maintainable. Use small servings of the following foods to enhance an already healthy snack or meal.

Food	Calories Serving	Fat (g)	Sugar (g)	Fiber (g)
Reduced-Fat Cheez-Its	130	4.5	0	1
Reduced-Fat Nilla Wafers	120	2	12	0
Reduced-Fat Honey Maid Honey Graham Crackers	140	2	8	2
Premium Whole Grain Crackers	70	2	0	1
Fat-Free Fig Newtons	90	0	12	1

Insider Tips

- The more snack foods you purchase, the more snack foods you are going to eat. Keep purchases to a minimum in this aisle in an effort to avoid overeating as much as possible.
- Use small portions to enhance an already healthy snack. One fat-free Fig Newton crumbled up makes a great topping for a healthy Greek yogurt. One whole-grain graham cracker can be a great place to add a teaspoon of peanut butter and banana slices.
- Use Wheat Thins Fiber Selects Five Grain crackers to make mini tuna-melt nachos. Simply place a layer of crackers on a microwave-safe plate. Top with low-fat tuna salad and shredded mozzarella cheese and melt

for about a minute. Enjoy by pulling one cracker away at a time.

- Pre-portion your crackers and cookies before your meal or snack begins. These two types of foods are probably the most difficult when it comes to portion control. If you already have a serving set aside, you are on your way to success.

Makeover Moments: Substituting whole grain, lower-sugar snacks for your old choices will have you feeling and looking different in no time. See how these little changes can positively impact your diet.

Food	Calories Serving	Sugar (g)	Fat (g)	Fiber (g)
2 Keebler Pecan Sandies*	170	7	10	1
100-calorie pack Keebler Pecan Sandies	100	6	4	3
Your savings	70	1	6	Gain 2

*Nobody can eat just two!

The next time you offer cheese and crackers as a snack, feel good about it by making these simple swaps.

Food	Calories Serving	Sugar (g)	Fat (g)	Fiber (g)
Ritz Crackers with 2 slices of Kraft American Cheese	200	1	13	0
Wheat Thins Fiber Selects with 1 Laughing Cow Lite Cheese Triangle	125	1	5.5	6
Your savings	75	0	7.5	Gain 6

Bottom Line

The super cool thing about changing the type of snack that you have is that it affects how you eat the rest of the day. People who snack on sugary, no-fiber snacks are always hungry. They are way more likely to grab that second handful of whatever is available. How you snack is the greatest influence on how you eat at meal time. Take extra time to create healthful snacks that you enjoy to set the tone for your day.

Bar None

The protein or granola bar has taken on celebrity status in our diets. We have grown to not only love their taste, but depend on their convenience. They are available in gluten-free, dairy-free, nut-free, and sugar-free formats. Some are acceptable for a snack and others could fill the place of an entire meal. Depending on how and when you intend to use nutrition bars, it is important to know what to look for next time you reach for the convenience of a protein or granola bar.

Key Food Facts

Fiber: I know you may be sick of me saying this, but if a bar is going to provide all of the nutrition as your snack it must have 3 grams of fiber. If your bar is intended to replace a meal, I am aiming higher and hoping for at least 5 grams of fiber per bar.

Protein: Unless you are on a protein-restricted diet, it is essential to incorporate protein each time you eat. But how much protein is enough to make you feel satisfied? Well, 1 ounce of protein, which is the equivalent of two egg whites or 1 ounce of chicken, has 7 grams of protein. As snacks, it would be ideal to find a bar that provided at least 7 grams of protein to help you stay full. A meal, however, should do more in the way of providing protein. Ideally, a meal replacement would have between 14 and 21 grams of protein per serving. Clif Builder's bars and Promax LS bars each fit the bill offering 20 grams and 18 grams of protein, respectively.

Fat: There will always be some fat in a nutrition bar. Oftentimes, the fat comes from nuts and whole grains in the bar. Other bars have added fat to create the candy bar–like coating you find on the outside of many bars. It is common for manufacturers to use palm kernel oil in the bars' coating. Palm kernel oil is a saturated fat and should be limited as much as possible. Try to find bars that have 5 grams of fat or less per bar.

Sugar: There are tremendous variations in the amount of sugar found in different bars. Certain bars have actual, visible dried fruit in them, which explains the source of the higher sugar content. When shopping for bars, I want to know the source of the sugar. For example, in a KIND bar, the sugar comes from the dried fruit. The same can be said for the Larabar, which has only whole ingredients. Limit added sugars in the form of cane sugar, honey, and syrups. The popular Nutri-Grain Cereal Bar's ingredient list has sugar or another type of sweetener as the top three ingredients in the filling, and the sixth ingredient in the crust. The 12 grams of sugar in each bar is not mind-boggling; however, knowing it is all added sugar is a bit of a turn off for me.

Pitfalls

- **Using a bar that does not have adequate nutrition for a meal.** The last thing you want to do is eat a bar with around 200 calories and feel hungry an hour later. Do not be afraid to add some extra food to your favorite protein bar to make a more complete and satisfying meal. For example, I will add two hard-boiled egg whites to my morning LUNA bar to keep me feeling full until lunch. If you need a bar to substitute for lunch, consider adding a bag of veggies, a piece of fruit, and a light string cheese to boost the nutritional value of that meal.

- **Do not sell yourself short.** Just because a bar offers one of the key ingredients, such as protein or fiber, does not mean that the bar as a whole is a great choice for your next meal. For example, a bar may provide 3 grams of fiber, which is terrific for a meal or a snack, but when you look for protein in that bar there are only 2 grams, making it extremely insufficient as a meal or snack replacement. Be sure to read labels completely to ensure the item meets all of your needs.

- **Unnecessary ingredients.** Avoid adding bars to your diet that are filled with unnecessary ingredients, including sugar alcohols. If a bar sounds too good to be true because it has zero grams of sugar, for example, be sure to keep reading. One bar I saw recently had 10 grams of sugar alcohols in it. That is enough sugar alcohols to cause GI distress in a large animal!

Everyday and Occasional Eats: In our busy and harried lives, there exists a need for nonperishable sources of balanced nutrition. In my clinical practice, I find bars to be exceptional options for student athletes and those who travel a great deal for work. Bars allow them to plan for extended periods of times when they will be away from a refrigerator or other dependable source of good nutrition. Based on your specific needs, the following bars may be options either every day or a few times a week when schedules are tighter.

Food	Calories Bar	Protein (g)	Fiber (g)	Fat (g)	Sugar (g)
LUNA bar	180	8	3	5	13
LUNA Protein bar	170	12	3	5	13
Clif Bar	240	10	5	6	22
Clif Builder's bar	270	20	4	8	20
MoJo bar	200	8	3	12	10
Larabar	240	5	5	13	22
Promax LS	220	18	14	7	9
KIND Bars	190	3	3	13	12
Kashi Cherry Vanilla Cereal Bars	120	2	3	3	9
Special K Protein and Fiber Bar	110	4	4	3	7
Kashi GoLean Crisp Bar	170	8	5	5	13
Kashi GoLean Roll	190	12	6	5	14
Kashi Chewy Granola Bar	120	5	4	2	8

Insider Tips

- Keep bars that you know agree with your stomach and your appetite on hand at all times. They eliminate any excuse you may have to visit the vending machine or simply going hungry.
- Most bars should cost around $1.00 each. Some grocery stores, including Whole Foods, offer a discount if you buy the whole box of one specific flavor. Once you find one you like, it may pay to stock up.
- I enjoy keeping bars in the refrigerator. It gives them a different consistency that makes the actual eating process take a bit longer and somehow makes the bar seem more satisfying.
- At Target, you can purchase mini versions of some of your favorite bars, including LUNA bars, in boxes of 10. These 80-calorie options might be a perfect partner for other healthful snacks, including fruit or yogurt.

Makeover Moments: By swapping a satisfying bar for one that hardly made the grade, you will notice that you feel full

Bar	Calories	Fat (g)	Protein (g)	Sugar (g)	Fiber (g)
Special K Bar	90	2	<1	7	3
Promax LS	220	7	18	9	14
Your gain	130	5	17	2	11

for significantly longer and that your energy level is improved as well. Check out the difference between these two bars in terms of their nutritional strength! I have many clients who eat "nutrition bars" for breakfast without realizing that the bar they are choosing does not have what it takes to be a meal. Sometimes more is better, and often in the case of protein bars, that is precisely the case.

Bottom Line

Eating whole food is best. For 200 calories, I would rather see you eat a three egg white omelet with two slices of light whole-grain toast and a teaspoon of peanut butter, but I know that is not always feasible. When time and convenience are factors, do not be afraid to choose a bar that not only tastes good but that is good for you.

Nutritional Inspiration from Around the World

Although unfamiliar foods can be a turn off sometimes, the truth is that there are a lot of hidden gems in the ethnic foods section of your favorite market. If you cannot locate these items at your corner store, check larger chains or specialty stores, or go online and check for retailers in your area.

Key Food Facts

Kosher Foods: Kosher is a designation assigned to foods that meet a certain certification required under Jewish law. These laws often have to do with how the food was prepared (how animals are raised and slaughtered) as well as how foods are combined together (kosher law does not allow for the combination of meat and dairy in the same meal). Furthermore, kosher foods are free from certain ingredients including pork, shellfish, and gelatin. Just because something is kosher does not mean it is healthy. Yet, if you have a kosher foods section in your market, there are a few secret food finds that fit into anyone's diet! Look for gefilte fish (in a jar), which is an excellent source for lean protein and a convenient way to fit fish into your diet. Also try bean and barley soup mixes and whole wheat Israeli couscous.

Mexican: Traditional Mexican foods have very much become a part of the American diet. With a fresh-Mex fast food restaurant popping up on nearly every corner, more people are growing to love the strong flavors of traditional Mexican cuisine. Look for amazing nutritional additions in the Mexican section of the market. Salsa, enchilada sauce, taco sauce, and vegetarian refried beans are some of my favorites. Mexican meals can be reformulated with healthy ingredients very easily because of their incorporation of high-quality products, such as plenty of vegetables, high-fiber beans, and lean meats.

Asian: Foods from Asian cultures are often low in calories and full of flavor. Look for low-calorie broth-based soups and healthful soy-based products. Low-sodium soy sauce is a calorie-free way to add a ton of flavor to just about anything, and one tablespoon of sweet and sour sauce has only 30 calories and a tremendous amount of zing! Sliced water chestnuts and rice noodles are also a must for healthy Asian-inspired salads and stir-frys.

Pitfalls

- Sodium: Just as with any canned, boxed, or jarred foods, items found in the international aisle are likely to be higher in sodium. If you are watching your sodium intake closely, be sure to check labels for sodium content in your favorite items.

- Boxed meals: Food manufacturers have started to sell entire meals in a box, including taco kits and Asian dinners. These meal combinations tend to be high in sodium, fat, and calories, with small serving sizes to boot.

Everyday and Occasional Eats: I rely heavily on certain items from this aisle to make my meals delicious and complete. Try adding one or two of the following to your usual menus for variety. Because of the higher sodium content of many of these foods, I would use them wisely, incorporating no more than one serving per day.

Food	Calories Serving	Protein (g)	Sugar (g)	Fiber (g)	Fat (g)	Sodium (mg)
Low-sodium soy sauce	15/Tbsp	1	2	0	0	550
Sweet and sour sauce	30/Tbsp	0	5	0	0	110
Whole Foods 365 Teriyaki Sauce	15/Tbsp	0	2	0	0	290
Sliced water chestnuts, canned in water	25	1	2	1	0	10
Instant miso soup	35	3	0	0	0	790
Manischewitz Split Pea Soup Mix	90/cup prepared	5	2	4	0	680
Rokeach Gefilte Fish	70/piece	9	0	0	2	420
Horseradish sauce	15/tsp	0	0	0	1.5	15
Vegetarian refried beans	90/½ cup	5	0	5	0.5	570
Salsa	9/2 Tbsp	0	1	0.5	0	198
Enchilada sauce	9/oz.	0	0.5	0	0	170

Insider Tips

- Use a teaspoon of horseradish sauce to add kick to your next turkey sandwich.
- Create a healthy Chinese chicken salad with chicken breast, sliced water chestnuts, fresh diced scallions, steamed broccoli and/or spinach, and 1 tablespoon of sweet and sour sauce.
- Enjoy healthy Mexican night at your house by creating vegetarian tacos using vegetarian refried beans, reduced-fat sour cream and shredded cheese, plenty of fresh veggies, and lots of salsa.
- Stir Fry! The easiest and most delicious way to incorporate large servings of vegetables into your diet. Use a small amount of olive oil and teriyaki sauce to make the simplest combinations of chicken, beef, shrimp, or tofu with vegetables.

Makeover Moments: Tacos are always a crowd favorite. Make them a healthy favorite by substituting some healthy ingredients for typically high-fat ones.

Food	Calories	Protein (g)	Fat (g)	Sugar (g)	Fiber (g)	Sodium (mg)
Hard taco with ground beef, sour cream, shredded cheese	260	14	17	2	2	500

continued on next page

Food con't	Calories	Protein (g)	Fat (g)	Sugar (g)	Fiber (g)	Sodium (mg)
Whole grain soft taco with vegetarian refried beans, reduced-fat sour cream and reduced-fat shredded cheese	200	16	2	2	14.5	500
Your savings	60	Gain 2	15	0	Gain 12.5	0

Bottom Line

The choices you make are cumulative. While the differences in each meal may be small and seem almost insignificant, the benefit of having healthy ingredients on hand adds up! If you make split pea soup on Monday in place of a creamy broccoli soup, you not only save calories at that meal, but also at the next meal when you enjoy the leftovers. I hope you find some international inspiration for new and exciting dishes the next time you visit your market.

Nuts about Nuts
& Dried Fruit, Too

What was once considered a nutritional "no-no" because of their high fat content is now heralded as the cure for all that ails you. Many nuts provide a natural source of healthy monounsaturated fats. These types of fats are heart protective because of their ability to raise HDL (good) cholesterol without raising total cholesterol. Nuts are also extremely satisfying because it takes a considerable amount of time for our bodies to digest and absorb the nutrition from fat-based foods. Studies have indicated that consuming one ounce of almonds an hour before a meal can significantly reduce the total amount of calories eaten at the meal. Nuts are nutrition powerhouses, full of iron, zinc, selenium, and B vitamins, including folic acid. Also high in antioxidants, nuts have the potential to be cancer-fighting missiles. Nuts should be used in small portions to enhance all sorts of meals and snacks.

Dried fruit and nuts are sort of "dating." They are paired

together in all sorts of trail mixes and salad topping kits. The magical combination of salty and sweet, crunchy and chewy just works! Dried fruit is dehydrated fruit that maintains all of the essential nutrients found in the original piece of fruit, except the water. The fiber, vitamins, and minerals contained in dried fruit are pretty close to the original, except the size is obviously considerably different. That is why cup-for-cup, dried fruit is drastically higher in calories than the original version. Dried fruit should be used sparingly as a topping on salads or fat-free yogurt.

Key Food Facts

Fat: Do not be surprised when you read the label on a container of nuts and see a lot of fat. On average, 1 ounce of nuts has 14 grams of fat, but that is not necessarily a bad thing. Nuts should be considered a "topping" for salads, yogurts, oatmeal, cereal, puddings, or stir fry. Choosing nuts as a standalone snack is likely to lead to overeating. While an ounce of nuts and all of their healthy fat is desirable, a cup of nuts is not. One cup of peanuts has 846 calories and 72 grams of fat, which is simply too much for anybody.

Sulfur dioxide is a chemical used to preserve and prevent microbial growth in certain dried fruit. Sulfur dioxide must be included on a nutrition label because of its potential negative effect on those who are either asthmatic or sensitive to sulfites. While there is no direct study that links human incidence of cancer to sulfur dioxide consumption, questions exist relative to its safety.

Sugar: Nuts are naturally sugar free, but dried fruit is not. Most dried fruit has about 30 grams of sugar per quarter cup. That is the equivalent of an apple and a half. Because of the relatively high-sugar content, dried fruit intake should be limited. The small serving size of common dried fruits, such as raisins, makes them an unsatisfying solo choice for most. Not to mention that those little sticky nuggets are not great for your teeth.

Pitfalls

- Portion Size: When consumers hear that something is good for them, like nuts in this case, they tend to overdo it. Only use nuts in small portions to enhance otherwise low-fat meals and snacks.
- False Appearances: Packages of dried fruit appear super healthy and although they are packed with vitamins, minerals, and antioxidants, their high sugar and calorie counts per small serving sizes make them an occasional food at best.

Everyday Eats: Latest recommendations from the USDA support including small servings of nuts each day. Check out the following list to see how your favorite nut stacks up. My favorites are almonds and pistachios because of their higher fiber content and relatively lower fat count. Studies have even indicated that eating nuts from the shell, rather than buying ones already out of the shell, leads to decreased intake. We are positively influenced by seeing the empty shells sitting in front of us, so we are less likely to continue eating.

Nut	Calories (per oz.)	Protein (g)	Total Fat (g)
Almond	169	6.3	15
Walnut	183	4.3	18.3
Peanut (actually a legume)	166	6.7	14
Cashew	163	4.3	13
Brazil nut	186	4	19
Macadamia nut	204	2	22
Pistacchio	161	6	13

Occasional Eats: The added sweetness of dried fruit can be enjoyed in small quantities throughout the week. Try sprinkling a few Craisins on your next salad or bowl of oatmeal. You do not need a large serving to enjoy a bit of sweetness.

Food	Calories (per 1/4 cup)	Sugar (g)	Fiber (g)
Raisins	123	24	2
Prunes	71	8.5	2.1
Apricots	78	17.4	2.4
Sunsweet Dark Chocolate-Covered Prune Bites*	190	20	3

*Enjoy one or two of these with a cup of coffee or tea after a meal. They make a nice mini-substitution for dessert.

Insider Tips

- Add a few slivered almonds at breakfast, lunch, or dinner. I like the slivered almonds because you get more bang for your buck. Add them to yogurt, cereal, oatmeal, salads, stir fry, or low-fat ice cream.

- Toast nuts on a baking sheet in the oven. Just watch them closely so they do not burn. Toasted nuts make a delicious and pretty salad topping. Bake a single row of almonds at 350° for 10-12 minutes. Toasted almonds can be stored in an airtight container for up to 3 months.
- Make your own healthy trail mix with low-fat popcorn, slivered almonds, and a small serving of dried fruit.
- Add a sprinkling of dried cranberries to your next salad. They look and taste beautiful!

Bottom Line

Just because something is good for you, it does not mean you should eat a lot of it. Use these healthy accents sparingly in your diet.

Seriously Talking Cereals

The way you start your day impacts everything—from your performance at work or school to your eating habits until bedtime. The business of breakfast cereals is an interesting one, as there are hundreds of options available, yet very few that are nutritionally sound. Paying attention to a few key tips can get your next bowl of cereal in tip-top shape.

Key Food Facts

Fiber: The only cereals that are really worth eating are those with at least 3 grams of fiber per serving. You may be very surprised when you read the labels on some seemingly healthy cereals, including Special K and Rice Krispies, and realize there is no dietary fiber in there. Without fiber, these cereals are likely to leave you hungry and unsatisfied. Some cereals have up to 14 grams of fiber per serving. For the average healthy adult, these may be a terrific choice. However, practice caution if providing such items to small children. That amount of fiber is likely to have a laxative effect and many kids do not want that feeling when they are at school. Typically, I would recommend 3–6 grams of fiber per serving for children.

Sugar: Was there a news bulletin that I missed where all Americans gathered together and told food manufacturers that they wanted to start their day with at least 3 teaspoons of sugar in their cereal? Well, if you have really looked at cereal labels lately the way that I do, you would surely think there had been such a decision. Whether they are filled with sugar-coated dried fruit or simply filled with added sugar, many common cereals are simply too high in sugar. Always look for cereals that have fewer than 10 grams of sugar.

When it comes to creating the perfect bowl of cereal, I have two main thoughts in mind—fewer than 10 grams of sugar and more than 3 grams of fiber. Obviously, beyond that, the more fiber and less sugar the better.

Calories: The calories in a serving of cereal range from 90 to 240 on average. It is important to note that serving sizes also vary greatly between cereals, so you are not always comparing apples to apples. Grape-Nuts, for example, has a ¼-cup serving size, while Cheerios assumes 1-cup servings. If you are attempting to keep total caloric intake within a certain range, you will likely want to choose cereals that offer servings for around 100 calories.

Fat: Generally, grains are naturally fat free, so by nature cereals should be low in fat. The only reason there should be fat in your breakfast cereal is if you are choosing a cereal that has healthy nuts in it. If there are no nuts or seeds, I would skip a cereal that has added fat.

Pitfalls

- Certain cereals seem healthy but are not. Whether it is their name or their packaging, it is easy to get roped into buying certain brands. Furthermore, many cereal companies are boasting the number of grams of whole grain on the face of their boxes, but this number does not necessarily mean that there is fiber in their products. Do not be seduced by the appealing packaging. Be sure to read labels before making a decision.
- Do not buy "kid's cereal" for your children. Turns out, nine out of 10 kid's cereals provide very little in the way of sound nutrition. Teach your kids to start their day with a less-sweet choice. My favorite, by far, is Quaker's Corn Bran Crunch. I've never had a client who did not like it.

Everyday Eats: Considering the large number of cereals on the market, there are very few that make the list of everyday eats. Hopefully this list will satisfy every eater at your breakfast table!

Cereal	Calories Serving	Sugar (g)	Fiber (g)	Fat (g)	Protein (g)
Quaker Corn Bran Crunch	90	6	4	1	2
Cheerios	100	1	3	2	3
Kix	110	3	3	1	2

Cereal	Calories Serving	Sugar (g)	Fiber (g)	Fat (g)	Protein (g)
Wheat bran flakes	100	5	5	.5	2
Oat bran flakes	110	6	4	1	3
Shredded wheat	170	1	6	1	6
Kellogg's Fiber + Antioxidants Cinnamon Oat	110	7	9	1.5	3
Nature's Path Sunrise Crunchy Vanilla	110	7	3	1	2
Hodgson Mill Steel Cut Oats	106	.7	3	1.8	3.5
Special K Protein Plus	120	3	7	1	10
Special K Multigrain Oats & Honey	100	8	3	.5	2
Life Crunchtime	110	7	6	1.5	2
Fiber One	60	0	14	1	2
Fiber One Honey Clusters	160	6	13	1.5	3
Fiber One Caramel Delight	180	10	9	3	3
Fiber One 80 Calories	80	3	10	1	1
Grape-Nuts	200	4	7	1	6
Kashi GoLean	140	6	10	1	13
Kashi Good Friends	160	10	12	1.5	5
Kashi Heart to Heart Honey Toasted Oat	120	5	5	1.5	3
Kashi Warm Cinnamon	120	5	5	1.5	4
Kashi Honey Sunshine	100	6	5	1	2
Kashi Cinnamon Harvest	180	9	5	1	6
Kashi Berry Blossoms	100	5	7	1	2
Barbara's Cinnamon Puffins	90	6	5.5	1	2
Quaker Lower Sugar Oatmeal	110	6	3	1.5	3
Steel cut oats	170	0	5	3	7
Better Oats Oat Fit	100	0	3	2	4

Occasional Eats: While I would prefer to see you choose from my list on a day-to-day basis, the following cereals are fun to include in different ways. I enjoy using them as toppings on frozen yogurt, mixed in with other healthy ingredients such as almonds and popcorn in a trailmix, or even as a topping on another super healthy cereal.

Cereal	Calories Serving	Sugar (g)	Fiber (g)	Fat (g)	Protein (g)
Apple Jacks	100	12	3	.5	1
Froot Loops	110	12	3	1	1
Peanut Butter Puffins	110	6	2	2	3
Frosted Mini Wheats	200	12	6	1	6
Bear Naked Fit Granola	120	4	2	2.5	4

Insider Tips

- Keep your opened cereal boxes on the shelf for up to two months. To avoid wasting too much cereal, choose one or two boxes at a time and use them until they are finished.
- Measure out a serving of cereal in your usual bowl. Once you know what that serving looks like in your bowl, you are more likely to stick to suggested serving sizes.
- Use cereal as toppings on any sweet treat, including frozen yogurt, Greek yogurt, fat-free pudding, or fruit salad. It is a relatively low-calorie crunchy snack!
- If you are used to a super sweet breakfast cereal, try mixing two brands at the beginning and slowly weaning off of the more sugary cereal until the

healthier option is all that is left.

- Try adding fresh fruit or slivered almonds to your next cereal bowl.
- Make an oatmeal and yogurt parfait. Mix 1 serving of oatmeal with a 4 oz. carton of fat-free yogurt for a breakfast that will not disappoint. I love adding chopped apples and a few nuts to the mix as well.

Makeover Moments: By changing the type and portion of cereal you have in the morning, you will completely transform your day! Check out these modifications.

Meal	Calories Serving	Sugar (g)	Fiber (g)
1 bowl of an average cereal with skim milk (1 cup)	340	32	4
1 bowl Kashi GoLean (1 cup) with skim milk (1 cup)	220	18	10
Your savings	120	14	Gain 6

Meal	Calories Serving	Sugar (g)	Fiber (g)
Quaker Instant Oatmeal	160	13	3
Quaker Lower Sugar Instant Oatmeal	110	6	3
Your savings	50	7	0

Bottom Line

Healthy habits begin at breakfast. The changes you will notice over the course of the day will astound you! Look for lots of fiber and less sugar to create a dream breakfast that will start you off toward eating healthy the rest of the day.

Who's Thirsty?

I would love to be able to make this the shortest section of the book by just saying, "Drink water!" However, with an entire aisle at the market dedicated to drinks, I suppose it requires a bit more explanation. Beverages account for roughly 10 percent of our daily caloric intakes, and many fingers have been pointing at the beverage industry over the last several years for single-handedly causing the obesity epidemic in this country. As a consultant to the Coca Cola Company (that produces more than 4,000 different beverages), I have been privileged to read nearly every study on the topic of beverages and health, and I feel comfortable expressing the concept of moderation when it comes to what is in your glass.

Key Food Facts
Sugar: Ideally, your drinks would not provide any sugar to your diet on a given day. Various beverages on the market

offer a wide range of sugar content. One 12-ounce can of regular soda can have 40 grams of sugar, while one 12-ounce glass of orange juice will have 31 grams of sugar. Remember, 1 teaspoon of sugar equals 4 grams of sugar. So a beverage that has 40 grams of sugar essentially contains 10 teaspoons of sugar. To put this in perspective, one cupcake with frosting has 50 grams of sugar; one fat-free Greek yogurt has 19 grams of sugar; one cup of Ben & Jerry's Cookie Dough ice cream has 50 grams of sugar; and one stick of cotton candy has 56 grams of sugar. While it is not up to me to decide how you spend your calories each day, consider making choices that limit your added sugar intake each day. If juice or soda is your favorite treat, enjoy them in smaller servings and less frequently to help keep your diet healthful.

Artificial Sweeteners: More and more, low- and no-calorie beverages are entering the market as alternatives to higher-sugar options. These types of drinks are typically sweetened with artificial sweeteners, including asparatame, NutraSweet, acesulfame K, Splenda, and Truvia (stevia extract). The safety of such ingredients is discussed at the beginning of this book (see "Planning for Perfection"). If calorie control is your main focus, choosing artificially sweetened beverages in place of sugar-sweetened ones is a good idea. Studies have shown that including diet sodas as part of a calorie-controlled diet can help dieters to reach their goal weight. Just be sure that diet drinks are not replacing essential water from your daily regimen.

Additives: Many drinks claim to raise you up, give you energy, fight cancer, improve vision, and make you stronger.

Waters with added vitamins, minerals, and phytochemicals are becoming more the norm than the exception. Drinks such as Vitamin Water Zero offer an array of different combinations of added nutrients to help give you a boost. "Are they good for you?" is the real question, and the real answer is "Maybe." I find them helpful with certain clients who just simply hate drinking water. Being able to offer them a caffeine-free, calorie-free source of hydration makes me happy. However, if you like drinking water, stick to it. It is the single best way to hydrate and rehydrate your body.

Electrolytes: These are key minerals that play a role in hydration status and blood pressure. We lose electrolytes when we sweat, vomit, or have diarrhea. Several drinks are marketed as electrolyte replacers for athletes. Unless you are exercising continuously for 90 minutes, replacement of electrolytes with a beverage is not necessary. This means that your little-leaguer who sat on the bench for 80 of the 100 minutes of his game does not need a Gatorade. Electrolyte loss can also be replenished with water and a balanced meal. A product relatively new to the market called Zico Coconut Water is also packed with electrolytes and can be used as a post-workout treat. Be sure to replace electrolytes if you are exercising intensely for 90 minutes or longer.

Caffeine: One cup of regular coffee has around 200 mg of caffeine. The U.S. government says that even pregnant women can enjoy up to 200 mg of caffeine each day as part of a healthy pregnancy. One can of regular soda has between 30 and 50 mg of caffeine and most energy drinks have around 80 mg of caffeine. A Grande cup of Starbucks' Pike Place coffee has 330 mg of caffeine per serving. For most people, the occasional serving of caffeine is fine and perhaps even beneficial. Caffeine has been shown to improve alertness and performance, as well as potentially play a role in prevention of dementia. Caffeine is one of the most studied ingredients in our food supply and its safety has always been upheld in studies. Many consumers report feeling dependent on caffeine during their day, yet there is no such thing as caffeine addiction. Use moderation when including caffeine-containing beverages in an effort to keep intakes near 200 mg per day.

Reduced Calorie or Light: When calories are on your mind, seek out reduced-calorie or light versions of your favorite juices. Food manufacturers replace about half of the usual sugar present in a drink with an artificial sweetener to maintain the taste you are used to having. If artificial sweeteners are not your thing, these beverages will be a pass. But if you do not mind the occasional serving of Splenda, these options can allow you to enjoy the occasional glass of juice.

Alcohol: While this is in no way an endorsement for alcohol consumption, I cannot talk about drinks without mentioning alcoholic beverages. If you are seeking out lower-calorie alcoholic options, consider choosing light beer in place of regular beer. Most light beers contain between 65 and 100 calories, while regular beers weigh in between 150 and 175 calories per 12-ounce serving. Wine typically contains around 100 calories per 4-ounce glass, with the exception of port wines that have 170 calories per 4-ounce serving. Keep in mind that a 4-ounce serving is half of a typical 8-ounce wine glass. Watch for higher sugar content on prepackaged drinks and mixers as well. Seek out low-calorie mixer options including club soda. If alcohol is part of your lifestyle, it should be enjoyed in moderation.

Pitfalls

- The obvious pitfall in the beverage aisle is overconsumption of full-calorie options. Add up the calories you obtain in your diet from drinks each day. If this amount is staggering to you, make a change. Swap water or club soda for full-calorie beverages several times throughout the day to decrease your calorie total.
- "Because it is juice, it must be good for me." Juice is not an essential part of our diet. It unfortunately provides a large number of calories—about 80 in a 4-ounce glass—and it tends to make us hungrier. It is a good idea to limit juice to special occasions, and if you have kids, I would encourage you to avoid making juice a regular part of their daily diet.
- Not drinking enough. On average, most adults need about 64 ounces of fluid each day. This number is increased if you exercise and sweat. Add one 8-ounce glass of water to your goal for each half hour that you sweat. If you work out for an hour in the morning, you need ten 8-ounce glasses of water that day. Do not wait until you are thirsty to drink. Once you are thirsty, your body has been dehydrated for about three

hours. Drink continuously throughout the day to prevent dehydration and to help keep your appetite in check. Quite often, human beings confuse thirst for hunger. We often look to food when, actually, we are thirsty.

Everyday Drinks: Choose from the following beverages for a natural source of hydration.

Drink	Calories 8 oz.	Sugar (g)	Caffeine (mg)	Artificial Sweeteners
Water	0	0	0	0
Crystal Light Pure Fitness Water additive	15	3	0	0
Club soda	0	0	0	0
Hint	0	0	0	0
Owater	0	0	0	0
Perrier	0	0	0	0

Occasional Drinks: Enhance your beverage selection from time-to-time with these low- and no-calorie drinks. If you are not concerned about artificial sweeteners, the following drinks could be part of a calorie-controlled diet each day.

Drink	Calories 8 oz.	Sugar (g)	Caffeine (mg)	Artificial Sweeteners
Crystal Light	0	0	0	Aspartame
Propel	0	0	0	Acesulfame potassium
Minute Maid Fruit Falls	5	<1	0	Sucralose
Aquafina Flavorsplash	0	0	0	Sucralose

continued on next page

Drink *con't*	Calories 8 oz.	Sugar (g)	Caffeine (mg)	Artificial Sweeteners
Vitamin Water Zero	0	0	0	Crystalline fructose and stevia extract
Fruit20	0	0	0	Sucralose
Crystal Bay	0	0	0	Sucralose and acesulfame K
Arizona Rescue Water	25	6	0	Stevia
Diet Snapple	0	0	0	Aspartame
SoBe Lifewater 0 calorie	0	0	0	Erythrit (sugar alcohol)
Diet Coke	0	0	45	NutraSweet
Zico Coconut Water	34	7	0	0
Twisted Water	38	8	0	0
G2	20	5	0	Splenda and acesulfame K

Insider Tips

- Club soda is a low-sodium, calorie-free beverage that can be a great substitute for regular soda or other full-calorie beverages. Add a spritz of any fresh fruit including orange, lemon, or lime to create just the right hint of flavor.

- Get yourself a great water bottle and carry it with you always. Staying hydrated will allow you to better pay attention to your hunger cues and likely make it easy to keep total caloric intake within acceptable levels.

Makeover Moments: You will not believe how much a shift in your daily beverage consumption can impact your week. See how changing certain habits adds up.

Remember, it only takes 3,500 calories to equal a pound of body weight. The habit of including full-

Drink Habit per day	Calories /week	Sugar (g)/week
2 cans regular soda	2,002	559
2 cans diet soda	0	0
Your savings	2002	559

calorie beverages multiple times a day can lead to a weight gain of almost 30 pounds a year.

Bottom Line

As I said at the beginning, drinking water is best. If that does not do it for you, seek out options that you feel good about, including smaller portions of full-calorie beverages or low- and no-calorie beverages whenever possible. Your body will thank you for the hydration!

Frozen Finds

Stock your freezer with healthy essentials to ensure that a healthy meal is always possible. Do not forget to put healthy leftovers into your freezer as well. It is a perfect way to save money and reduce food waste. It is always a good idea to check calories per serving to determine if the food is a good choice. A frozen meal should have more than 200 calories in it or you will still be starving when the meal is over. A frozen waffle, on the other hand, should be lower in calories and a serving of frozen vegetables will have very few calories.

Key Food Facts

Fiber: Almost every item that is worth buying in the freezer aisle will have fiber in it. Fiber should be present in your waffles, frozen vegetables, frozen entrees, and frozen side dishes. Look for at least 3 grams/serving.

Fat: Watch for added fats in your favorite frozen finds.

You do need fat in your diet, and I would expect you to get some fat in certain foods, such as an entire dinner or frozen meat substitutes. You do not need added fats in foods such as waffles or pancakes, or fruits and vegetables, so read labels and ask yourself if the fat that is in the dish is acceptable and necessary. A good rule of thumb is to keep fat to less than 30 percent of total calories, or three grams of fat per 100 calories.

Sodium: Frozen vegetables tend to be much lower in sodium than canned varieties. The sodium content can get high, however, in frozen meals, as salt is included as a preservative and flavor enhancer. Look for sodium content of less than 600 mg per serving.

Pitfalls

- **Too convenient to be true.** Frozen entrees seem so easy. They have protein, grains, and vegetables all wrapped into one little package. Lean Cuisine even offers calorie-controlled options that don't break the calorie bank. The only real problem is that the serving provided in that box may not be satisfying to you as a meal. In order to keep calories in check, portions are often extremely small in healthy frozen entrees. Be sure to include plenty of fresh vegetables with your next frozen meal so that you are not left feeling hungry just a short time later.
- **To the exclusion of all else.** Choosing primarily frozen foods takes the fun out of cooking and experimenting with new flavors and ingredients.
- **Poor choices.** I know I said there are a lot of healthy

choices in the freezer aisle, but there are also a lot of unhealthy ones. Watch for supersize pizzas, extra-large beef dinners, butter-laden veggies, and chocolatey breakfast items. Even some of the organic frozen entrees lack any nutritional merit.

Everyday and Occasional Eats: I always make a trip down the freezer aisle to grab essentials that keep my freezer stocked for simple, healthy meals.

	Calories Serving	Protein (g)	Fat (g)	Fiber (g)	Sugar (g)	Sodium (mg)
Breakfast Foods						
Eggo Low-Fat Whole Grain Waffles	140	5	2.5	3	3	390
Kashi GoLean Blueberry Waffles	170	8	3	6	4	300
Van's Gourmet 97% Fat Free Waffles	180	5	2	5	4	306
Vitalicious Egg n' Cheese Vitasandwich with Veggies	150	14	2	7	3	340
Vitalicious Pumpkin Spice Muffin Top	100	3	1	8	8	110
Morningstar Farms Vegetarian Sausage Patty	80	10	3	1	0.5	260
Cedarlane Egg White Frittata	180	13	7	5	4	300

	Calories Serving	Protein (g)	Fat (g)	Fiber (g)	Sugar (g)	Sodium (mg)
Vegetables						
All frozen fresh vegetables	Varies	Varies	Varies	Varies	Varies	Varies
Green Giant Broccoli in Low-Fat Cheese Sauce	60	2	2.5	2	3	460
Green Giant Niblets Corn in Butter Sauce	100	3	1.5	1	5	280
Green Giant Healthy Weight Frozen Vegetables	90	5	2.5	5	3	230
Pizza						
Lean Cuisine Deep Dish Roasted Vegetable Pizza	320	16	5	3	6	480
Kashi Roasted Vegetable Stone Fired Pizza	250	14	9	4	3	630
Amy's Light & Lean Italian Vegetable Pizza	280	13	6	4	6	560
Entrees						
Lean Cuisine Spa Cuisine Salmon	210	15	5	5	2	590
Van De Kamps Parchment Bake Tilapia	80	13	0	1	0	350
Tabatchnick Minestrone Soup	100	5	1.5	4	3	320

	Calories Serving	Protein (g)	Fat (g)	Fiber (g)	Sugar (g)	Sodium (mg)
Entrees						
Dr. Praeger's Spinach Pancakes	80	2	4	2	0	190
Cedarlane Lentil Vegetable Soup & Samosa Wrap	230	10	6	5	4	480
Cedarlane Veggie Burrito	260	13	1	7	2	490
Amy's Low-Sodium Vegetable Lasagna	290	15	8	4	8	340
Morningstar Farms 3-Bean Chili	270	20	4	16	6	800
Veggie Burgers and Other Meat Substitutes						
Morningstar Farms Garden Vegetable Patty	110	10	3.5	3	1	360
Morningstar Farms Chick'n Patty	140	8	5	2	1	590
Morningstar Farms Chick'n Strips Meal Starters	140	23	3.5	1	1	500
Boca Flame Grilled Burger	120	14	5	5	0	380
Boca Ground Crumbles, made with natural ingredients	60	13	.5	3	0	270

Insider Tips

- Add volume and satisfaction to any frozen entrée by mixing in plenty of fresh or frozen vegetables. For most of us, the fewer than 300 calories provided by healthy entrees is not satisfying enough to be dinner. A large salad or cut-up veggies to go along with it should help the meal stretch a bit longer.
- If you have kids, teach them how to make a frozen veggie burger for part of a snack. These are great sources of nutrition, safe, and are ready in less than two minutes. Make a sandwich on a high-fiber sandwich thin for a snack that is just 200 calories.
- Use healthy low-fat cheesy vegetables as a terrific topping for a baked potato.
- Top a low-fat, whole-grain waffle with fresh fruit and use nonfat yogurt in place of syrup.

Makeover Moments: Each frozen entrée is unique. Just because it seems like it might be the same does not mean that it is. Look at the difference between the two following fettuccini Alfredo frozen entrees. Which one would you choose?

Meal	Calories Serving	Fat (g)	Protein (g)	Fiber (g)	Sugar (g)	Sodium (mg)
Stouffer's Fettuccini Alfredo	610	34	18	5	7	1,030
Lean Cuisine Fettuccini Alfredo	300	6	16	3	5	660
Your savings	310	28	−2	−2	2	370

Bottom Line

Stock your freezer with essentials to ensure that a healthy meal is always possible. Do not forget to put healthy leftovers into your freezer as well. It is a perfect way to save money and reduce food waste!

Dairy Delight

I recently attended a conference sponsored by the United Dairy Industry of Michigan. As part of our afternoon activities, we took a field trip to a dairy farm. I was admittedly a bit apprehensive about spending the afternoon among cattle. As it turned out, I was completely blown away by the experience. The chief veterinarian explained how they calculate the nutrition in the cattle feed each day to meet the specific needs of the animals. They clearly spent more energy planning meals for the cattle than most parents spend on configuring their own child's diet.

The dairy products that are so readily accessible at any market have origins at dairy farms across America. These products offer a unique blend of carbohydrate and protein with varying amounts of fat. They are incredible sources of micronutrients including calcium, potassium, phosphorus, protein, vitamins A, D, and B12, riboflavin, and niacin. Keep reading to see how incorporating low-fat dairy can be easy and delicious!

Key Food Facts

Fat: Dairy products come in all sizes. Some are full-fat varieties that may taste good but are not necessarily good choices on a regular basis. These full-fat dairy items, including whole milk and full-fat yogurts and cheese, have saturated fat in quantities that are out of line with current diet recommendations. Whole milk contains 3.25% fat. The good news? There are plenty of reduced-fat and fat-free dairy options from which to choose. Reduced-fat dairy items are often identified as either "reduced fat," "2%," or "1%" on the packaging. These products, on average, cut the amount of fat in a product at least in half. For example, a glass of whole milk has 148 calories and 8 grams of fat, while a glass of 2% milk has 122 calories and only 4.8 grams of fat, and a glass of skim milk has 80 calories and 0 grams of fat.

My favorite reduced-fat dairy products are cheeses. Reduced-fat shredded cheese looks, tastes, and melts just like full-fat cheese, without all the grease and fat. You should not have a hard time finding several reduced-fat cheeses at the market. Many fat-free dairy products also exist. My favorite fat-free dairy items include skim milk, fat-free yogurt, pudding, and nonfat ice cream. I'll be honest, switching from full-fat dairy to reduced-fat or fat-free takes a bit of time to get used to. Give the process six weeks, and you will be happy you did.

Calories: Just as the fat in various dairy products differs from one product to the next, so do the calorie levels. Look for all sorts of low-fat cheese snacks for 60 calories or less. Reduced-fat string cheese, Mini Babybel Light, Light Laughing Cow Cheese Wedges, and 2% or Fat-Free Kraft Singles all provide protein and calcium in calorie-controlled portions that meet everyone's needs.

Artificial Sweeteners: While I make every attempt to limit artificial sweeteners in my own diet and the diets of my clients, I always recommend yogurt that is artificially sweetened. The difference in calories and grams of sugar between full-sugar and artificially sweetened yogurts is astounding. Some full-sugar yogurts have near 30 grams of sugar, while artificially sweetened ones hover between 10 and 15 grams. The benefits of eating yogurt, in my clinical mind, outweigh the small amount of artificial sweetener you may get in your daily yogurt. Certain brands are sweetened with aspartame and NutraSweet (Yoplait Light and Dannon Light & Fit), while Dannon Activia Light is sweetened with Splenda and acesulfame K, and Yoplait 100 calorie Greek Yogurt is sweetened with acesulfame K.

Calcium: We rely heavily on dairy products to help us meet our calcium needs each day. Calcium requirements differ by age. Each serving of dairy provides between 250 and 300 mg of calcium. For most adults, that means you would need to include four to five servings of low-fat dairy in your diet each day to meet your calcium needs. For many consumers, that is simply too many calories to consume from dairy. Discuss the importance and safety of taking a calcium supplement with your physician if your daily dairy intake does not quite get you to your calcium goal.

Age	Calcium (mg/day)	Vitamin D (IU/day)
4–8	800	200
9–18	1,300	200
19–50	1,000	200
51–70	1,200	400
70+	1,200	600

Lactose Free: Lactose is a natural sugar found in milk products. Certain people have a difficult time digesting lactose, causing gassiness, bloating, and diarrhea that is quite uncomfortable. These symptoms are different and should not be confused with a milk allergy. It is estimated that up to 70 percent of adults have some degree of lactose intolerance. If you have noticed symptoms of intolerance when you choose certain dairy products, look for lactose-free varieties. Lactaid brand serves up a whole line of lactose-free dairy products to choose from including cottage cheese, yogurt, milks, and ice cream.

Pitfalls

- Overconsumption: Cheese is yummy and so are yogurt and ice cream. It is important to watch serving sizes when it comes to choosing dairy products. Try to purchase calorie-controlled portions including Kraft 100-Calorie Pack cheeses, Sargento Reduced-Fat String Cheese, Kraft 2% singles, Light Laughing Cow Cheese, or Mini Babybel Light cheeses to help keep overeating to a minimum. Yogurt, puddings, and 2% cottage cheese are also available in single-serving cups of less than 100 calories.
- Concerned about taste: I have had so many clients tell

me that reduced-fat cheese or skim milk tastes like water or that they would rather not have any dairy products if they cannot have the "real thing." It only takes about 6 weeks for taste buds to adjust to a new way of eating. Do not sell yourself short by avoiding this important and healthful food group.

Everyday Eats: Low-fat dairy should be part of your diet every day unless you are vegan or have an allergy or intolerance to milk. The following favorites are great sources of protein and match up well with fruit or veggies to make a balanced snack or meal.

Food	Calorie	Fat (g)	Protein (g)	Sugar (g)	Sodium (mg)
Skim milk (8 oz)	90	0	9	12	125
Sargento Reduced Fat Shredded Cheese (0.5 oz)	40	3	3.5	.5	90
Sargento Reduced Fat String Cheese (1 stick)	50	2.5	6	0	160
Light Laughing Cow Cheese (1 wedge)	35	2	2.5	1	260
Mini Babybel Light Cheese (1 circle)	50	3	6	0	160
Philadelphia 1/3 Less Fat Cream Cheese Spread (1 Tbsp)	35	3	1	1	70
Kraft 2% Singles (1 slice)	50	2.5	4	2	290
Breakstone's 2% Cottage Cheese (4.4 oz)	90	2.5	12	4	400

Food	Calories	Fat (g)	Protein (g)	Sugar (g)	Sodium (mg)
Kozy Shack No Sugar Added Rice Pudding	70	1	4	5 (also has 3 g fiber)	120
Fat-free ricotta cheese (1/4 cup)	50	0	5	2	65
Reduced-fat feta cheese (1 oz)	58	3.8	5.8	0	392
Lifeway Light Farmers Cheese (1 oz)	24	.9	2.8	.9	9
Reduced-fat sour cream (1 oz)	39	3	1	<1	20
Fat-Free Reddi-Wip (2 Tbsp)	5	0	0	1	0
Dannon Activia Light (4 oz)	70	0	4	8	65
Yoplait 100 Calorie Greek Yogurt (5.3 oz)	100	0	13	7	55
Simply Go-Gurt (1 tube)	70	.5	2	10	30
Dannon Light n' Fit (6 oz)	80	0	5	11	80
Yoplait Light (6 oz)	100	0	5	14	85

Occasional Eats: These decadent dairy delights are fun to include once or twice a week as part of a balanced diet.

	Calories	Fat (g)	Protein (g)	Sugar (g)	Sodium (mg)
Cheese					
Light Muenster cheese slices (1 oz)	80	4.5	9	0	120
Kraft 2% Reduced-Fat Cheddar Cheese (1 oz)	90	6	7	0	240
Laughing Cow ⅓ Less Fat Cream Cheese Spread	45	4	2	<1	140

	Calories	Fat (g)	Protein (g)	Sugar (g)	Sodium (mg)
Puddings, Ice Creams, and Non-Dairy Frozen Goodies					
Jello 100 Calorie Fat Free Pudding (4 oz)	100	0	2	17	190
Jell-O Sugar Free Pudding Cups (3.7 oz)	60	1.5	2	0 (has sugar alcohols)	180
Skinny Cow Low-Fat Ice Cream Sandwich	140	1.5	4	15 (3 g fiber)	135
Blue Bunny No Sugar Added Fat Free Vanilla Ice Cream (½ cup)	80	0	4	5 (2 g sugar alcohol)	70
So Delicious Neapolitan Low-Fat Non-Dairy Ice Cream Mini Sandwich	90	2	2	8	70
Edy's Slow Churned Yogurt Blends (½ cup)	90	0	3	14	45
Edy's No Sugar Added Fruit Bars	30	0	0	2	0
Edy's Slow Churned No Sugar Added Creamy Ice Cream	100	3	3	3 (4 g sugar alcohol)	35
Spreads					
Smart Balance (1 Tbsp)	45	5	0	0	85
Earth Balance	100	11	0	0	120
Best Life Spread	60	6	0	0	100

Insider Tips

- Use 2% cottage cheese as a high-protein cheesy sauce for cooked rice or pasta. Simply add into recently drained pasta or rice and mix to make a healthy mac n' cheese alternative. Cottage cheese makes a delicious topping on toast as well. Sprinkle with a little cinnamon and Truvia (if you like) and you will have a low-calorie snack with a high-calorie taste.

- Non-fat yogurt and skim milk are the perfect ingredients for a smoothie. The 1-1-1 recipe is a cinch. 1 cup skim milk, 1 cup nonfat vanilla yogurt, and 1 cup frozen fruit come together perfectly in a blender. Add in high-fiber cereal for an added crunch!

- Spread Light Laughing Cow Cheese on everything. Use it instead of mayo on sandwiches, on slices of fruit for a snack, on whole grain crackers, or mixed into warm pasta. The company itself recommends melting Laughing Cow and mixing with salsa to make a cheese dip for veggies or whole grain chips. The opportunities are endless!

- Add whole-grain cereal as a topping on a Yoplait 100 Calorie Greek Yogurt for the perfect snack.

- Use reduced-fat sour cream in dips and recipes in place of the full-fat version. Nobody will ever know the difference.

- If you are lactose intolerant or allergic to milk, seek out dairy alternatives including almond, soy, or rice-based products to help you meet your calcium needs.

- Limit the use of spreads on vegetables and breads. You will get used to enjoying meals without the added calories and fat.

Makeover Moments: Take the leap into the world of low-fat dairy and see what you have been missing!

Food	Calories Serving	Fat (g)	Protein (g)	Sugar (g)	Fiber (g)	Sodium (mg)
Dannon Fruit on the Bottom Yogurt	150	1.5	6	26	0	105
Yoplait Greek 100 Calorie Yogurt	100	0	13	7	0	55
Your savings	50	1.5	**Gain** 7	19	0	50

Now you do not just have to dream about dessert!

Food	Calories Serving	Fat (g)	Protein (g)	Sugar (g)	Fiber (g)	Sodium (mg)
Ben & Jerry's Chocolate Chip Cookie Dough Ice Cream (½ cup)	270	14	4	25	0	60
Edy's Slow Churned Chocolate Fudge Brownie Ice Cream (½ cup)	120	3.5	3	14	1	40
Your savings	150	10.5	−1	11	+1	20

Bottom Line

Each serving of dairy that you switch to reduced fat or fat free will end up saving you about 40 calories, 4 grams of fat, and 15 mg of cholesterol. These tasty changes will help to get the scales "mooooving" in the right direction.

Eggstravaganza

I love talking about eggs with my clients. Did you know that eggs are the perfect source of protein? They earn a 1.0, or perfect score, on the Protein Digestibility Corrected Amino Acid Score, which is used by scientists to determine the adequacy of various protein sources. Each egg has about 60 to 80 calories, depending on its size. It is also has 7 grams of protein, which is almost all contained in the white part of the egg. That is the same amount of protein as in one ounce of chicken or meat. Each egg white has only 17 calories, all of which is derived from protein, and is completely fat- and cholesterol-free. So can we all stand up and bow to the awesome egg white and all of its uses in our daily diets.

Key Food Facts

Antibiotic-Free: Somewhat of a "non-term" in the egg world. No eggs are ever injected with antibiotics according to the Egg Nutrition Center. If a hen requires antibiotics, its eggs are not used for human consumption under FDA regulations.

Shell Color: Brown eggs and white eggs are created equal. Their nutritional value is identical.

Cage-Free or Free-Roaming: Eggs produced by hens that have free range of an indoor facility with access to food and water at all times.

Free-Range: Eggs produced by hens that have access to the outdoors as well.

Vegetarian-Fed: Eggs produced by hens that are fed vegetarian diets. This label is not specifically regulated by the USDA.

Hormones: Not used in the production of any shelled eggs in the United States.

Shelf Life: Eggs can be kept in the refrigerator for up to five weeks from the date of purchase.

Nutrient-Enhanced: Eggs that are produced by hens fed a special diet. This may lead to increases in the amount of lutein, omega-3 fats, and vitamin E in each egg.

Organic: Eggs that are produced in accordance with the USDA's organic standards.

Grade: Grades range from AA, which is the highest, to A and then B. These grades refer to the quality of the egg and not the size of the egg.

Pitfalls

- Exceeding Cholesterol Limits: Each whole egg has 213 mg

of cholesterol. The American Heart Association recommends keeping cholesterol intake to less than 250 mg per day. This makes egg yolks, in my opinion, a food to use sparingly.

Everyday Eats: These variations of the whole egg are a wonderful way to add fat-free protein to any meal.

Food	Calories	Protein (g)	Fat (g)	Cholesterol (mg)
Egg white	17	3.6	0	0
100 Percent Whites (¼ cup)	30	6	0	0
Egg Beaters (¼ cup)	30	6	0	0
Egg-Land's Best Hardcooked Peeled Eggs (only white)	17	3.6	0	0

Occasional Eats: The whole egg is a nutrient-dense food that may fit within your diet goals occasionally. Here are the stats!

Food	Calories	Protein (g)	Fat (g)	Cholesterol (mg)
1 Large egg	70	6	4	213

Insider Tips

- Use hard-boiled egg whites for everything! Make a healthy egg sandwich in the morning by placing the whites of two hard-boiled eggs on an Arnold Sandwich Thin, top with a pinch of reduced-fat shredded mozzarella, and melt in the microwave or toaster oven. Add a slice of fresh tomato for a real treat!

- Use two egg whites in the place of one whole egg in most recipes.
- Make egg-white omelets and egg-white frittatas that are sure to please. Add in your favorite veggies and low-fat cheese and you will have a meal that keeps you full for hours.

Makeover Moments: Substitute two egg whites for one whole egg for recipe magic!

Food	Calories	Protein (g)	Fat (g)	Cholesterol (mg)
1 large egg	70	6	4	213
2 egg whites	34	7.2	0	0
Your savings	36	+1.2	4	213

Bottom Line

Throw yourself an eggstravaganza each and every day by including heart-healthy egg whites in a multitude of ways. Make whole eggs an occasional food in order to keep your cholesterol in check.

Part Three

Putting It
All Together

The next time you go grocery shopping, you will clearly be the smartest one in the store. You have a plethora of information to help guide you down any aisle of any market across the country. It is a good idea to plan for perfection by organizing your thoughts into weekly lists. This will make cooking healthy meals a snap.

Weekly Shopping Lists: Use the following sample week to provide you inspiration in the kitchen. Come on guys, I can't make it any easier!

Sunday	
Breakfast:	Corn Bran Crunch, skim milk, 2 hard-boiled egg whites
Lunch:	Tuna salad with low-fat mayo, veggies for salad, 1 Arnold Sandwich Thin
Snack:	1 Yoplait 100 Calorie Greek Yogurt, 15 almonds
Dinner:	Chicken breast, asparagus, baked sweet potato
Snack:	1 pear

Monday

Breakfast:	2 slices Aunt Millie's Light Potato & Fiber Bread, toasted 2 slices low-fat cheese
Lunch:	Turkey deli meat, 1 Flatout Light, Hummus, cut up veggies, fruit
Snack:	1 banana, 1 Tbsp peanut butter
Dinner:	Turkey meatballs & spaghetti, squash with marinara sauce
Snack:	1 grapefruit

Tuesday

Breakfast:	1 Thomas' Bagel Thin with light cream cheese, 2 hard-boiled egg whites
Lunch:	Greek salad, light dressing, Arnold Pocket Thin
Snack:	1 apple, 1 light string cheese
Dinner:	Steak fajitas, 1 Flatout Light for tortilla
Snack:	Low-fat microwave popcorn

Wednesday

Breakfast:	1 LUNA bar, 1 cup skim milk
Lunch:	Egg white omelet with veggies and light cheese, 2 slices light toast
Snack:	Veggies and hummus
Dinner:	Grilled salmon, roasted Brussels sprouts, wheat pilaf
Snack:	1 Skinny Cow Ice Cream Treat

Thursday

Breakfast:	Kashi Good Friends Cereal, skim milk, 1 hard-boiled egg white
Lunch:	2 % cottage cheese, ½ cantaloupe, whole grain crackers
Snack:	1 Yoplait 100 Calorie Greek Yogurt, ¼ cup Bear Naked Fit Granola
Dinner:	1 lean hamburger, whole grain hamburger bun, large salad, balsamic dressing
Snack:	Berries with Reddi-Wip

Friday

Breakfast:	Egg white and low-fat cheese sandwich on an Arnold Sandwich Thin
Lunch:	Bowl of soup, low-fat chicken or tuna salad, fruit
Snack:	Celery with peanut butter and raisins
Dinner:	Baked chicken, lentil pilaf, steamed spinach
Snack:	100 calorie chocolate pudding

Saturday

Breakfast:	1 bagel thin with light cream cheese and smoked salmon
Lunch:	Salad with walnuts, dried cranberries & grilled chicken or tuna
Snack:	1 small bowl of cereal
Dinner:	Whitefish, baked potato, low-fat coleslaw
Snack:	Edy's Fruit Bar

Week 1 Grocery Lists

Breads

Arnold Sandwich Thins
Arnold Pocket Thins
Aunt Millie's Light Potato
& Fiber Bread
Flatout Light
Thomas' Bagel Thins

Meats/Poultry/Fish

Chicken (white meat)
Ground white meat turkey
Lean turkey deli meat
Sirloin (for fajitas)
Lean ground beef
Salmon (½ lb/adult)
Whitefish

Grains

Near East Wheat Pilaf
Near East Lentil Pilaf
Orville Redenbacher 94%
Fat Free Butter Popcorn

Produce

Brussels sprouts
Sweet potato
Spaghetti squash
Peppers and onions
Asparagus
Lettuce
Tomato
Carrots
Spinach
Baking potato
Shredded cabbage
Celery
Cantaloupe
Berries
Grapefruit
Pear
Apple
Avocado

Cereals

Quaker Corn Bran Crunch
Kashi Good Friends
Bear Naked Fit Granola

Canned Goods

Progresso Macaroni &
Bean Soup
Beets (for Greek salad)
Chick peas
(for Greek salad)

Dairy
Skim milk
Reduced-fat sour cream
Light string cheese
Yoplait 100 calorie
Greek Yogurt
Low-fat sliced cheese
Low-fat shredded cheese
Low-fat feta cheese crumbled
2% cottage cheese
Reddi-Wip topping
Jell-O 100 calorie pudding

Freezer
You could buy frozen vegetables in lieu of fresh if you prefer
Skinny Cow Ice Cream Sandwich
Edy's Fruit Bar

Other
Hummus
Walnuts
Almonds
Dried cranberries
Peanut butter (Jif Omega-3 or Reduced Fat)
Fajita spice packet mix
Salsa

Eggs
Egg-land's Best
Hard-boiled Eggs
100% egg whites (in carton)

Turkey Meatballs and Spaghetti Squash

Ingredients

1 lb. ground white meat chicken or turkey

½ cup Italian flavored bread crumbs

¾ tsp garlic powder

½ tsp ground black pepper

½ tsp oregano

1 28-oz can whole tomatoes or 1 jar tomato sauce

1 spaghetti squash

Olive oil

Crushed garlic

Preheat oven to 400°. Prick all over the outside of the spaghetti squash with a fork and place on a baking sheet. Bake until soft to the touch (about 1 hour). Halve the squash crosswise, scoop out seeds, and scrape strands with a fork into a bowl. Season squash with salt, pepper, 1 teaspoon olive oil, and crushed garlic to taste.

Mix remaining ingredients in a bowl with your hands and shape mixture into meatballs. Place the meatballs in a large nonstick skillet and cook with 1 Tbsp of olive oil over medium heat until they are golden brown on the outside, roughly 5 minutes. Add 1 28-oz can whole tomatoes or 1 jar tomato sauce. Bring tomatoes to boil and reduce heat to a simmer and cover. Cook for 15 minutes. Uncover and cook for 15 more minutes.

Serve with meatballs and sauce over the spaghetti squash. Sprinkle with reduced-fat parmesan cheese. Makes 4 servings.

Nutritional Information

Serving: ¼ recipe

Calories: 336

Carbohydrates: 24 g

Fiber: 5 g

Protein: 20 g

Fat: 12 g

Fajitas

Prep Time: 10 minutes

Cook Time: 10 minutes

Ingredients

1 pkg. McCormick Fajita Seasoning Mix

2 Tbsp. oil, divided

1 lb. boneless skinless chicken breasts or boneless beef sirloin, cut into ½-inch strips

1 medium onion, cut into thin strips

1 medium bell pepper, cut into thin strips

¼ cup water

8 high-fiber flour tortillas (6-inch) or Flatout Lights

Assorted Toppings: reduced-fat shredded cheese, salsa, reduced-fat sour cream, guacamole, sliced tomatoes.

Heat 1 tablespoon of oil in large skillet on medium-high heat. Add meat; cook and stir 3 minutes or until no longer pink. Remove from skillet. In same skillet, heat remaining 1 tablespoon oil. Add onion and bell pepper; cook and stir 3 to 5 minutes. Return meat to skillet.

Stir in water and seasoning mix. Cook and stir 3 minutes or until heated through.

Spoon into warm tortillas. Serve with toppings, if desired. Makes 8 servings.

Shopping to Travel: Before you board your next plane, train, or automobile, run down this travel shopping list for nutritious, nonperishables that travel just as well as you do.

- Jif To Go (individual packs of peanut butter; you cannot take a large container of peanut butter on an airplane. The airlines consider it a liquid.)
- Blue Diamond Almonds (chocolate mint is my favorite)
- Apples (travel well without refrigeration)
- LUNA bars (or other protein bars that you know you enjoy and tolerate well)
- Healthy cereal in resealable plastic bags.
- Popped low-fat popcorn
- Roasted seaweed or kale chips if you can find them packaged. (Trader Joe's has excellent roasted seaweed.)
- Sugar snap peas can last for a while outside the fridge. They are not moist, making them convenient for snacking on the go.
- Water (it is really easy to become dehydrated when traveling). Be sure to buy a bottle of water or bring an empty bottle with you and fill it at a drinking fountain, both after you pass through security.

Shopping for One: Shopping for one can be really fun because you can buy exactly what you want! By incorporating leftovers from dinner into next-day lunches, you can stretch your dollar and your efforts. Check out these helpful tips to make grocery shopping an empowering process for you.

- Turkey burgers for dinner crumble easily for a high-protein topping on salads the next day. They last in the fridge for two days, so make enough to last for the next couple of lunches.
- Roasted vegetables are the most amazing salad toppers

ever. They also are terrific in a sandwich, so be sure to add them to your turkey roll up or tuna salad.

- Use a portion of higher cost foods, such as avocado or mango, in Mexican dishes for dinner and use the remainder as a salad topper the next day.
- Use leftover rice and chicken to create a healthy grain salad for the next day.
- Freeze foods in single portions for easy reheating.

Shopping for the Crew: As the number of mouths to feed increases, so does the cost and frequency of grocery shopping. Whether there are 3 or 13 of you, it may be time for you to embrace the concept of shopping more often. Running into the store two to three times a week for 15 minutes each time, instead of spending two hours on a Sunday, will help you to keep healthy foods on hand all of the time.

- Shop for three days at a time. With a lot of people running in a lot of different directions, it is difficult to predict what should be for dinner a week ahead of time. This also helps to ensure you are getting the freshest products.
- Do not give into food jags. As long as there are no food allergies or intolerances, make one dinner each night that everyone is welcome to enjoy. Avoid becoming a short-order cook, making several meals each night.
- Buy bulk items of foods you know your family will use up each week.
- Let your kids get involved in this process. Have them search health-based web sites such as eatingwell.com

for recipes using their favorite ingredients. When they help to plan meals, they are significantly more likely to try and enjoy them.

- If you have a crockpot, use it! If you do not have one, you should really think about getting one. The crockpot must have been invented by a busy parent who was sick of making dinner. It is simple to put together complete meals in the crockpot in the morning and enjoy them at the end of a crazy day for dinner. Try this crock pot recipe to get you started!

Creamy Chicken and Vegetables

Prep Time: 20 minutes
Cook Time: 7 hours, 30 minutes
Total Time: 7 hours, 50 minutes
Ingredients
    4 pounds chicken, skin & fat removed,
       cut into serving pieces
    1 tsp. salt
    ¼ tsp. pepper
    2 Tbsp. olive oil
    2 lbs. sweet potatoes, halved
    1 (16-oz.) package baby carrots
    1 onion, chopped
    3 cloves garlic, minced
    14-oz. can low-sodium vegetable or chicken broth
    1 cup plain Greek yogurt or So Delicious dairy-free
       Greek yogurt

3 Tbsp. Dijon mustard

3 Tbsp. honey

3 Tbsp. whole grain flour

1 tsp. dried thyme leaves

Preparation:

Sprinkle chicken with salt and pepper. Heat olive oil in large skillet and brown chicken.

In 4–5 quart slow cooker, place potatoes, carrots, and onion. Top with chicken. Pour broth over all. Cover crockpot and cook on low for 7–8 hours until chicken is thoroughly cooked and vegetables are tender.

In small bowl, stir together Greek yogurt, mustard, honey, flour, pepper, and thyme until well blended. Stir into mixture in crockpot and turn heat to high. Cook for 15–20 minutes, stirring occasionally, until thickened. Serves 8.

Coupons: The cost of grocery shopping for the average family of four varies between $120 and $220, depending on the budget. By clipping coupons and joining your market's frequent shopper plans, you are likely to put a bit of a dent in that total.

- Join your market's frequent shopper program. There are discounted prices on a variety of items each week.
- Subscribe to your local newspaper. You can save a good amount of money on coupons clipped from the paper.
- Did you know many grocery stores will accept competitor's coupons? Try offering your 10 percent

off coupon from ABC grocery store to DEF grocery store and see what happens.

Let Your Phone Do the Shopping If you have a smartphone, search your app store for coupon apps.

Grocery IQ offers easy access to online coupons, as well as an easy place to make grocery lists by typing or scanning UPC codes on your favorite items.

Grocery Pal points you in the direction of sale items at your local supermarkets and superstores including Wal-Mart, Target, Publix, and Kmart.

Pepperplate.com allows you to store recipes in your smartphone easily. It will also help you to effortlessly find recipes online and import them into your library. This app is unique as it also converts each recipe into a shopping list for your convenience.

Meal Planning by Food on the Table (www.foodonthetable.com) offers weekly menus and meal planners, including healthy kid's recipes.

The Five Minute Shop: Keep several quick dinner shopping lists on hand at all times. This will allow you to be in and out of the market in five minutes with a complete meal in hand.

Five-Ingredient Meals

Baked Chicken Dinner

Chicken breasts (one to two 3-piece packages)
1 bottle low-fat French dressing

1 box onion soup mix

1 bag baby carrots

1 box wheat pilaf

Rinse chicken and pat dry. Place chicken and carrots in a glass baking dish.

Cover with French dressing and onion soup mix.

Bake at 350° for an hour or more until done.

Cook wheat pilaf in boiling water during last 35 minutes according to package directions.

Stir Fry

Tofu, Chicken, Shrimp, or Beef

Two packages cut-up Asian vegetables (usually available in fresh produce section)

1 package brown rice

1 bottle stir-fry sauce or teriyaki sauce (low-sodium if you prefer)

Olive oil

Use small amount of olive oil to cook protein (tofu, chicken, shrimp, or beef) in a cast iron skillet or wok.

Add in vegetables and sauce, and cook until vegetables reach desired consistency.

Cook rice according to package (when a recipe calls for butter or oil, feel free to omit or use sparingly).

Seasoned Salmon

Salmon (1 lb./2 people)

1 Tbsp dried thyme

½ tsp paprika

½ tsp cayenne pepper ground

Cooking spray

Preheat oven to 350° and apply cooking spray to one side of aluminum foil piece large enough to wrap over the entire piece of fish.

Place salmon on foil and season with other ingredients. Cover salmon completely and bake for about 20 minutes.

Five-Ingredient School Lunches

Pita Pockets

Arnold Pocket Thins (both whole-grain and Italian herb are excellent)

1 lb. of lean deli turkey (or other protein source)

Individual hummus packs

Carrots

Apple

Cheese Please

Breakstone's 2% Cottage Cheese in a 4-pack

1 cantaloupe or pineapple

Celery stalks

Light ranch dressing

Individual popcorn bags

Crackers Galore

Wheat Thins Fiber Selects 5 Grain Crackers

Mini Babybel Light Laughing Cow Cheese (any flavor your prefer)

Yoplait 100 calorie Greek Yogurt

Berries (could be delicious on the yogurt or on the side)

Sugar snap peas

Online Resources: Many of us have the internet in our pocket 24 hours a day on our smartphones. There are many reliable places to visit that can also provide excellent support for your healthy lifestyle.

www.usda.gov

www.fda.gov

www.eatingwell.com

www.calorieking.com

www.nutritiondata.com

Bottom Line

Grocery shopping is something most of us have to do. I'll admit it is not romantic or particularly thrilling on a regular basis. I'll even admit that most of the time I do not look forward to going to the market, but there is something so incredibly satisfying in knowing that you are doing right by yourself and your family by providing the fuel you all need to excel. There is even something exhilarating about opening a stocked refrigerator and seeing all of the different colored fruits and vegetables.

The fundamentals of this book are intended to help guide you to better health by changing the way you think about food. Remember to always go back to the basic principles outlined here if you are confused and overwhelmed. New products will continuously flood the marketplace each week, but the rules by which we determine if something is good for us do not change much. Read labels and use common sense. When in doubt, shop the perimeter of the store seeking out whole foods that are not processed or refined in any way. Good health through good food is an obtainable and realistic goal for everyone. Here's to your good health!! (This is where we clink our glasses of club soda with lime ;))

Index

calories of, 69, 71
everyday eats, 71
fiber content of, 69
"gluten free," 70
occasional eats, 71
serving size of, 70, 71
sodium content of, 69
week 1 grocery lists, 212
and weight loss, link between, 68–69
Brown rice pasta, 133
Brown rice vs. white rice, 133
Buckwheat, 133

C
Caffeine
daily intake limit for pregnant women, 182
in drinks, 182–183
Calcium
American diet and, 24
in dairy products, 197–198
Calcium supplements, 24
Caloric intake, 21
calculating, 36
Calorie-controlled diet, 69, 181, 185
100-calorie packs, 152, 154
200-calorie packs, 152
Calories in serving of
alcoholic beverages, 183–184
bread, 69
cereals, 175
condiment aisle, 109
condiments, 109
crackers and cookies, 152
dairy products, 196–197
dried fruits, 170
eggs, 204
freezer aisle, 188
juice, 184
spaghetti sauces, 140
spreads, dressings, and marinades, 109
Canned food industry and bisphenol A, 102
Canned foods, 102
attempting to limit, 105
beans, 104
calcium disodium EDTA in, 103
canned vegetables and soups, 104–105
fats in, 103–104
making over choice of, 105–106

moderation concept and, 105
MSG in, 103
sodium content of, 103
substituting fresh/frozen vegetables
for, 105
week 1 grocery lists, 212
Carbohydrate foods, guidelines for
purchasing, 41
Carbohydrates
definition of, 11
fiber-full, 14–16
fiber-less (See Refined carbohydrates)
recommended daily intake of, 11
types of, 11
Carbs. See Carbohydrates
Cardiovascular health, fats impact on, 20–21
Carrots, sugar content of, 60–61
Cereals
calories in, 175
everyday eats, 176–177
fat in, 175–176
fiber in, 174–175
makeover with, 179
measuring out a serving of, 178
mixing two brands of, 178–179
oatmeal and yogurt parfait, 179
occasional eats, 178
shopping guidelines for, 38, 176
sugar in, 175
as toppings on sweet treat, 178
week 1 grocery lists, 212
Certified Humane, 96
Cheese-based sauces, 140
Cheese please, 222
Cheeses, 196, 200
Laughing Cow, 202
Chips
regular vs. baked, 149
substitute for
cooked seaweed, 148
homemade kale chips, 148
nachos, 149
veggies, 149
Cholesterol. See also HDL cholesterol;
Total cholesterol
AHA on daily intake of, 206
in eggs, 205–206
and heart-healthy fats, 20–21

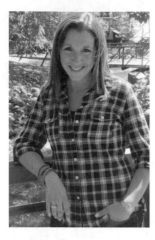

Julie Feldman, MPH, RD

Julie Feldman, MPH, RD, traveled her own path to arrive in the field of nutrition and dietetics. As an overweight child, she began a health transformation at the age of 12. Now, as a practicing dietitian for the past 13 years, she continues on her journey, educating and empowering both children and adults on their own quests to better health.

Julie graduated from the University of Michigan in 1996 and went on to U of M's School of Public Health to obtain her MPH degree in Human Nutrition. Julie works in her own private practice based in Farmington Hills, Michigan, where she provides counseling and consulting services to individuals, families, teams, and corporations. She thoroughly enjoys spreading the message of sound nutrition, appearing frequently on television and in print as a nutrition expert.

Julie currently lives in Farmington Hills, Michigan, with her husband and three children. She practices what she preaches, enjoying daily exercise, cooking often, and participating in many forms of physical activity with her kids. Her children love that she is a dietitian, except when she says they cannot have ice cream two nights in a row.